JOSEPH A. LAYDON JR.

THE GETTYSBURG PROGRAM

WHAT YOU DON'T KNOW MAY BE KILLING YOU –

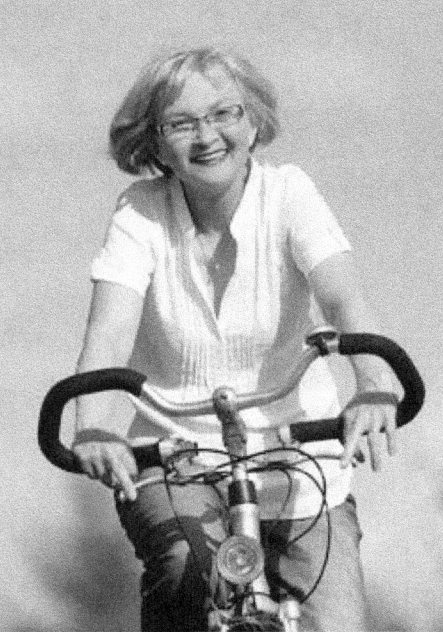

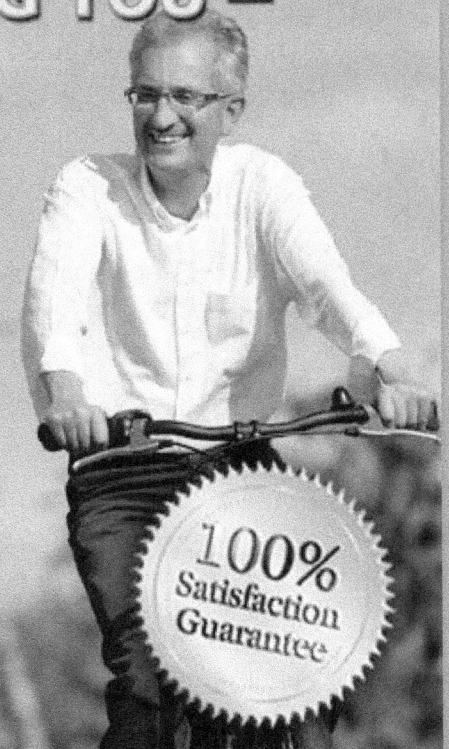

100% Satisfaction Guarantee

YOUR COMPLETE GUIDE TO BETTER HEALTH AND VIBRANT LIVING!

(SMALL 100+ PAGE VERSION)

The Gettysburg Program!
(short version)

What You Don't Know May Be Killing You -
Your Complete Guide To Better Health And Vibrant Living!

Thank you for getting your own **The Gettysburg Program.** This book (small version – 40,062 word count) is based on my *"intensive research"* and healthy experiences.

This book is designed to expose you to not only healthy eating but alternative ideas, alternative healthcare practices, and serious every day threats to your health at home and work.

OK, check out the Table Of Contents where you'll get a good idea of how The Gettysburg Program can benefit you today for your healthy future.

Published By Joseph A. Laydon Jr.

Website: http://www.survivalexpertebooks.com

E-Mail: wwwsurvivalexpert@yahoo.com

MOST IMPORTANT NOTE: This Gettysburg Program IS THE SMALL VERSION (143 - pages). I put this Book together as an introduction to the full version which is 620 pages and approximately 220,458 word count.

I highly encourage you to get the full version which clocks-in at 620 pages and a word count of approximately **220,458!** Click this link to go to my website to read more details about **The Gettysburg Program – What You Don't Know May Be Killing You. Your Complete Guide To Better Health And Vibrant Living!**

Copyright

IRISAP DISCLAIMER STATEMENT

Dedication

This Book is dedicated to YOU and all those other good folks out there that KNOW there are alternative heathcare practices that work where conventional medicine of drugs and surgery fail.

Each year in the US of A alone, approximately 500,000 Americans die of cancer. Each year in the US of A alone, approximately 500,000 Americans die of heart disease.

And each year THOUSANDS more Americans die from strokes, diabetes, autoimmune diseases, degenerative diseases.

The author feels Americans shouldn't rely soley on conventional medicine cause the American healthcare system is broken, unreliable, and money driven.

I encourage you to read this entire book. I know you'll like this Book. Therefore I highly encourage you to get the **FULL VERSION of The Gettysburg Program** (775 pages - approximately 220,458 word count).

Thank you for showing your wise interest in this Book.

PS Let me tell you this: *"There are approximately 300,000 plants on the Earth, uncountable species of insects, many small game, big game, and marine & aquatic that live & cover more than 75% of the Earth's surface. And the outright and undisputed CURE for every minor malady to sickly killers is within those 1,500,000+ species of plants, insects, small & big game, and within all that life in fresh and salt water throughout the Earth. One day, an international institution will finally be founded and this will be the beginning of the end for all sickness on the Earth for man and critters! Thus a beginning for a utopic world."*

Table Of Contents

Contents

"DO NOT SEND ME ANY MONEY. I Will Send You Any   03 Of 10 Survival Tricks Of

INTRODUCTION

Welcome to *"The Gettysburg Program – What You Don't Know May Be Killing You. Your Complete Guide To Better Health And Vibrant Living!"* This Special Report is the <u>small version</u> and focuses on alternative healthcare practices from eating the best healthy foods, and many other alternative healthcare practices and exposing daily threats to your health.

This Book gives you 26 Sections of abbreviated (small version) healthy reading and addresses multitudes of alternative healthcare practices besides the conventional medicinal practices of drugs and surgery.

I highly encourage you to read this Special Intelligence Report more than a few times to better understand all the related data.

And I highly encourage you to get the **full version of the Gettysburg Program** (approximately 200,000 word count).

Sincerely,
Joseph A. Laydon Jr.

CONGRATULATIONS for having the desire to change your healthy future for the better! Once you read this entire book you will never be the same unhealthy person again! Don't believe me, read the book. OK, you paid for information so here we go. You will NEVER be the same unhealthy person again!

Each year more than 1,400,000 Americans die of the HEART DISEASE, CANCER, and STROKE and I'm not covering deaths from many other degenerative diseases, infectious diseases... Each day three out of every four deaths in the United States occur as a result of cardiovascular\heart disease like heart attacks and stroke. Americans are spending billions of dollars on exercise machines, worthless fad diets, and health care (medical operations to aid in weight loss and to cure ailments and diseases). Diseases caused by the processed foods we eat have too much sugar, too much salt, far too much saturated fat, too much cholesterol, and the lack of vital nutrients.

Every second of every day, you're exposed to alcohol, EMF (Electromagnetic Fields), dermatophagoides, exhaust fumes, pesticides, pollution, processed foods, preservatives, poor nutrition, stress, ETS (Environmental Tobacco Smoke), toxins, x-rays, and VOCs (Volatile Organic Chemicals).

These environmental hazards and your own lifestyle choices cause arthritis, bruising, cancer, heart disease, lack of energy, liver damage, mental deterioration, poor circulation, premature aging, and susceptibility to sports injuries.

The continual bombardment of stress, environmental pollution, food processing, and an unhealthy lifestyle allows your body to be more susceptible to disease which determines your state of health.

Your two pound immune system with its trillion cells from the lymphocytic family and 100 million trillion antibodies is supposed to defend your body from all foreign infectious invaders from a simple scratch to AIDS to many chronic degenerative diseases like aging, arthritis, heart disease, and cancer.

The food you eat, the water and other liquids you drink, the air you breathe, your lifestyle and what you think affect how healthy you are right now and in the future. There are multitudes of toxic chemicals, pesticides, pollutants, and toxins in our environment. Americans eat far too much processed food that is lacking in vital nutrients but are rich in sugar, salt, saturated fat, and cholesterol. Americans are continually stressed from everyday living. Our immune system isn't performing to its peak, meaning we are not as healthy and healthy looking as we could be. GIVE your body the inherent chance to heal itself with proper nutrition, supplements, and avoiding the continual threats of everyday life from poor nutrition, environmental threats, and your own lifestyle!

The purpose of this book is to educate you to be a healthier and healthier looking person. Being healthier will reflect your attitude and performance. This book will inform you about a wide variety of conventional and alternative health care information, as well as alternative medical practice, unknown hazards to your health and their conventional and alternative remedies. This book will give you hundreds of resources (addresses and phone numbers) to refer to for additional information and resources for alternative medicine as well as conventional medicine. TAKE ADVANTAGE of the information in Section 25 you paid for it!

I'm giving you healthy information that is supposed to be *"none of your business!"*

YOU HAVE THE RIGHT TO THIS INFORMATION. ONLY YOU CAN CHOOSE TO BENEFIT FROM THIS IMPORTANT AND REVEALING INFORMATION. KEEP IN MIND THAT THIS BOOK IS NOT FOR SELF-DIAGNOSIS NOR A SELF-PRESCRIPTION TO HEALTH. ONLY A QUALIFIED PHYSICIAN OF YOUR CHOICE CAN DIAGNOSE AND PRESCRIBE THE PROPER MEDICATION AND THERAPIES IN YOUR FAVOR TO A HEALTHY PRESENT AND HEALTHY FUTURE. IF YOUR DESIGNATED PHYSICIAN FAILS TO AT LEAST LOOK INTO THE HEALTHY INFORMATION PROVIDED WITHIN THIS BOOK AND CALLS IT B.S., THEN YOU MAY WANT TO THINK ABOUT GETTING ANOTHER PHYSICIAN THAT CARES MORE ABOUT YOU AND LESS ABOUT YOU AS A SOURCE OF REVENUE!

Did you know that in the last 20 years, 24,000 babies have been born with spina bifida and anencephaly because their mothers were deficient in folic acid the first four weeks of pregnancy. Why? Refined food is one reason (removal of even a speck of folic acid is disastrous) and the other reason is ignorance; not on the part of the pregnant mothers but on the medical establishment.   The health establishment is at fault for not educating not only doctors but all women especially women who require folic acid before and during pregnancy. Lack of timely medical research not only for folic acid but a myriad of other supplements (you'll soon read about in this book as well as free requested information from Section 25) hinders millions of Americans from quality life they deserve but don't get because of ignorance.

If there is the slightest hint that something besides a drug or scalpel could remedy a symptom or disorder, then the medical establishment must at least look into it and so should you!
THE LACK OF NEEDED HEALTHY INFORMATION AND RESOURCES WHETHER CONVENTIONAL OR ALTERNATIVE IS THE REASON FOR THIS BOOK!

If you're a World Class athlete or even a jogger, exercise is absolutely great but it's not the only answer to vibrant health nor is it enough. World Class Athletes have dropped dead in their tracks and they've exercised, worked-out, and ran countless miles! People who have exercised every day for decades, like those in the military, have dropped dead in their tracks! Why? What's in that food you eat, the water or liquids you drink, the air you breathe, and the content of your thoughts? I'll tell you all about these matters and what to do about it later.

In 1971, the United States Department of Agriculture (USDA) conducted a study and estimated that dramatic savings from health care would take place if diets could be improved. Some examples include reduction in heart and vascular problems by 25 percent, reduction in the number of people with arthritis by 50 percent, and reduction of the number of deaths and acute conditions from cancer by 20 percent. This study was from 1971 and the estimates are considered quite low!

The number of people involved in providing health care in the United States is over 5 million - making it one of the largest industries in the country and costing more than $1.5 billion a day (1989). No other country spends such enormous amounts on the health of its citizens (actual or per capita). U.S. citizens SHOULD BE THE HEALTHIEST PEOPLE IN THE WORLD BUT WE ARE NOT!

In the following 26 Sections, I'm going to reveal healthy information you should have known about a long time ago and information that is SUPPRESSED or shunned as B.S. by those that like the traditional drug and scalpel treatment! Why are more and more doctors looking into Alternative Medicine versus conventional medicine? Better yet, why are more and more folks like you and I turning towards Alternative Medicine? The following 26 Sections of healthy reading will answer this question.

SECTION ONE - Eat The Right Stuff

According to the American Medical Association and the National Academy of Science, consume at least five servings of fruits and vegetables a day for good health and to avoid cancer, heart disease, and other health risks. According to the U.S. Surgeon General, 68% of all disease is diet related. The Standard American Diet is out of balance, consisting of far too much saturated fat, sugar, sodium, and cholesterol. Fiber is lacking as is regular exercise and supplements of Vitamins, minerals, and other health supplements that you'll read about that have benefited multitudes of Americans and healthy people throughout the world. So what foods are good to eat? This first section EAT THE RIGHT STUFF will get you off to realizing the benefits of EATING THE RIGHT STUFF. Some of these same foods have literally reversed diseases and afflictions and are recommended to patients who suffer from a variety of maladies and diseases by leading doctors throughout the U.S. and just about every country in the world.

You must SEE Vita-Mix TNT in Section 25. Here are some healthy quotes:
* *"Eating less fat can reduce the risk of colon, prostate, and breast cancer."* - National research Council, *"Diet and Health"* (1989)
* *"The single most influential dietary change one can make to lower the risk of these diseases is to reduce intake of foods   high in fats and to increase the intake of foods high in complex carbohydrates and fiber."* - The Surgeon General's Report on Nutrition and Health (1988)

WARNING SIGNS that your present diet may be your unhealthy enemy are: food allergies, colds, constipation, flu, hemorrhoids, high blood pressure, indigestion, obesity, sinus infection... Let's start with those healthy vegetables.

To botanical historians the *"Anticancer Cruciferous Twelve"* all have flowers that resemble a crucifix or cross; thus cruciferous. They all share common chemicals that can counteract some of the destruction from carcinogens.

Broccoli	Kale
Brussels sprouts	Kohlrabi
Cabbage	Mustard
Cauliflower	Radish
Cress	Rutabaga
Horseradish	Turnip

Now let's discuss some amazing health benefitting vegetables!

VEGETABLES

Artichokes: A medium artichoke furnishes only 53 calories and is low in fat. Artichokes contain calcium, iron, phosphorous, niacin, Vitamin C, magnesium and potassium. Studies in Japan, Switzerland, and Russia provide evidence that artichokes lower cholesterol. Cynarin which is a drug derived from artichokes lowers cholesterol. Cynarin is well known to be *"liver protective"* in both animal liver cells and living animals.

Russian scientists noted that the edible parts of artichokes were noted to exert an anti-inflammatory activity in dogs.

In 1969, French scientists were so successful in using artichoke extract for treating liver and kidney ailments, they took out a patent on it!

Artichokes are available throughout the year but their freshest peak production are the Spring months. Artichokes are consumed by eating the tender part of the leaves. Draw the leaf between the teeth to eat the tender meaty portion. Discard the leaf. Eventually, you'll get to the very delicious heart or bottom of the tasty artichoke. It's very tasty and VERY HEALTHY for you!

Asparagus: Asparagus is undoubtedly one of the most healthiest foods on Earth! Asparagus provides no fat, no cholesterol, and hardly a trace of sodium. Four spears of asparagus provides only 13 calories. Asparagus is so low in calories that you would have to really eat huge amounts of it to gain weight.

Asparagus is full of three food based nutrients that help in the defense of cancer. These elements are Vitamin A, Vitamin C, and the mineral selenium which is excellent for its antioxidant properties. Asparagus also contains small amounts of cholesterol-lowering fiber. Asparagus is ideal for heart-healthy menus.

According to studies at the University of California and Mount Sinai School of Medicine in New York, regular asparagus consumption demonstrates lower rates of cancer and heart disease.

Broccoli: Did you know broccoli is America's favorite vegetable? One stalk of cooked broccoli furnishes only 45 calories and .2 grams of fat. According to the U.S. Department of Agriculture, broccoli is the leading source of dietary fiber, packed with potassium, provides Vitamin B, low in fat and even calcium (for strong bones and teeth). Broccoli is noted for its cancer-fighting properties (chemoprotectant). Broccoli may be the number one cancer-fighting vegetable. Researchers at Johns Hopkins of Medicine in Baltimore have isolated a 'chemoprotectant' substance called sulforaphane which has been identified in broccoli. Sulforaphane may be the most potent cancer protecting agent to date! Sulforaphane actually stimulates the body's cells to produce cancer fighting enzymes. Other cancer-fighting chemicals are indoles, carotene and Vitamin C. Broccoli is noted to help flush fat out of your system.

Brussels Sprouts: One-half cup of raw Brussels sprouts provide only twenty calories while one-half cup of cooked Brussels sprouts provides 30 calories. A member of the cruciferous vegetable family (broccoli, cabbage, cauliflower), Brussels sprouts can fill you up and help you lose weight. A cooked cup of this tasty treat is rich in Vitamin C, provides a good share of Vitamin A, iron, potassium, riboflavin, and rich in protein. Brussels sprouts are very low in fat and sodium and provide fiber.

Brussels sprouts are a good bet to inhibit cancer, especially colon and stomach cancer. According to Dr. Saxon Graham's 1978 study in Buffalo, New York, Brussels sprouts emerged (along with cabbage and broccoli) as outstanding in saving lives from colon cancer!

According to a study in Norway, eating more cruciferous vegetables, including Brussels sprouts may suppress the precancerous growths in the colon called polyps in which cancer initially surfaces. Brussels sprouts and other cruciferous vegetables may also cut the risk of bladder, esophageal, lung, rectal, stomach and rectal cancer!

Brussels Sprouts Tasty Recipe!

MOST IMPORTANT NOTE: Here's my quick recipe for Brussels sprouts. I normally don't eat or like the taste of Brussels sprouts till I cooked em' up this way.

Ingredients: 24 Brussels sprouts, sharp knife, frying pan, coconut oil, bowl, fork, sea salt and wooden spoon.

Step 01: Take a frying pan put it on one of your burners at medium heat.

Step 02: Immediately spoon-out 05 good oversized scoops of coconut oil (will be semi-solid at room temperature) and put them in the frying pan and wait till the coconut oil starts sizzle.

Step 03: Procure 24 Brussels sprouts and cut off the base (stalk) of each of them. Then remove 03 or 04 outer leaves (debris) and place them in the frying pan.

Step 04: Every couple minutes or so, gently stir the Brussels sprouts in the frying pan with your wooden spoon till they are all golden brown.

Step 05: Remove to Brussels sprouts to a bowl and sprinkle them with sea salt. Fork-in and enjoy with a cold bottle of beer.

Note: I tried cooking the Brussels sprouts with other oils, but coconut oil is the tastiest and it's a Medium-Chain Triglyceride (MTC) meaning it helps you burn fat far better than other oils that aren't MTCs.

Cauliflower: Cauliflower is a bit more costly, but worth it when it comes to your health. One cup of raw cauliflower furnishes only 31 calories, provides a good source of Vitamin C (one cup equals 100% of RDA), low in sodium, and low in fat. Cauliflower is noted to help flush fat out of your system. Cauliflower is one of the vegetables recognized by the Committee on Diet, Nutrition and Cancer of the National Academy of Sciences as one of the best bets for preventing cancer! Cauliflower has established itself as being high on the list of anticancer vegetables.

A close cousin to cabbage, broccoli, and Brussels sprouts - all of these vegetables are linked to lower cancer rates, especially of the colon, rectum, stomach, and possibly the bladder and prostate. Norwegians who eat their fair share of cauliflower (along with broccoli, Brussels sprouts, & cabbage) have fewer and smaller precancerous polyps of the colon.
According to a study by Dr. Lee Wattenberg, laboratory animals were fed cauliflower and then given powerful carcinogens like nitrosamines. The animals that ate cauliflower did not readily develop cancers as those animals that didn't eat cauliflower.

Kale: Kale is super vegetable as a potential preventative of several cancers including lung cancer. Noted to be one of the richest of all green vegetables in cartenoids (anticancer agents) and a highly nutritious food, spinach has 36 milligrams of cartenoids per 100 grams. However, an equal amount of kale has more than twice the amount of cartenoids (78 milligrams). Too bad kale isn't a popular food item in the United States and Western countries.
A study in Singapore noted that kale, along with common dark-green leafy vegetables like Chinese mustard greens, has significantly diminished the risk of lung cancer!

Mushroom: At this time few medicinal benefits from the popular and common mushroom in the United States have been researched and proved. However, four Oriental mushrooms (shiitake, oyster, enoki, and tree) contain compounds that can stimulate the immune system, inhibit blood clotting, and retard the development of cancer. Japanese scientists have analyzed the medicinal qualities of mushrooms, especially the shiitake mushroom which is popular in the United States.

Scientists note that some mushrooms possess properties that may strengthen the immune system against a variety of infections, cancer, and possibly autoimmune diseases like rheumatoid arthritis, polyarthritis, and multiple sclerosis.

The most common and best-studied mushroom with the greatest therapeutic qualities is the shiitake, also known as *"golden oaks"* in the United States. In 1960 Dr. Kenneth Cochran of the University of Michigan launched a study of the shiitake mushroom. He discovered this mushroom contained a compound called lentinan, a long-chained sugar called a polysaccharide, which has a strong antiviral potential that stimulates the immune system functions! Shiitake stimulates the immune system to produce more interferon, which is a natural defense agent against viruses and fighting cancers. The shiitake compound, lentinan, has proved itself in fighting cancers. It has been tested in leukemia patients in China and on breast cancer patients in Japan.

In follow-up Japanese tests, lentinan was found to be far more effective against influenza viruses than a powerful antiviral drug called amantadine hydrochloride. More tests found that lentinan is a broad-spectrum killer of various viruses.

Consuming shiitake could help lower blood cholesterol and even block the bad effects of highly saturated fats. In one study, a group of thirty healthy young women drove their blood cholesterol down by an average of 12 percent by simply eating 3-ounces of shiitake each day for a week.

Could shiitake counter the effect of fat in the diet? In another study, one group ate two ounces of butter every day for a week; their cholesterol went up 14 percent. Another group ate the same amount of butter every day for a week, but added three ounces of shiitake. Guess what? Their blood cholesterol dropped 4 percent instead of rising 14 percent (non-eaters of shiitake)!

Onion: A 1/2 cup of raw onions provide only 27 calories and are inexpensive. Onions are used in just about every dish imaginable, from appetizers to main courses to soups to even jellies. Onions can be eaten raw, they can be pickled, sauteed, deep fried, boiled, or steamed. Onions help boost the good cholesterol which is HDL (High Density Lipo-proteins), lower total blood cholesterol, slow down blood clotting, thin the blood, kill bacteria and may even counteract against some allergic reactions.

Dr. Victor Gurewich, professor of medicine at Tufts University, prescribes and tells his patients to *"Eat onions."* Dr. Gurewich notes that raw, strong onions elevate critical HDL-type blood cholesterol. The typical therapeutic dose is only 1/2 a medium-size raw onion - or equivalent juice - each day.

Dr. Gurewich says that is usually enough to *"dramatically raise"* HDLs (good cholesterol) an average of 30 percent in about 03 out of 04 heart disease patients! In a few cases, HDL levels have doubled or tripled on the onion regimen! He says that raw onions work best because cooking lessens or destroys the onion's power to raise HDLs. Raw or cooked onion works as a natural anticoagulant to help prevent life-threatening blood clots that may cause heart attacks and strokes!

According to a study in India, test participants were purposely fed fat-intensive meals that raised their cholesterol to dangerous levels, thus increasing the risk of blood clots. The participants were then given only two ounces of onion, which was added to their diet, and their cholesterol levels were quickly brought within safe limits!

Onions may be a potential source of possible cancer antidotes because of their concentrated sulfur compounds that are able to turn off cell changes preceding cancer growth. Researchers at the M.D. Anderson Hospital and Tumor Institute have isolated propylsulfide in onions that in tests blocked enzymes needed to activate a potent cancer-causing substance.

Researchers at Harvard School of Dental Medicine discovered that putting onion extract on cultures of oral cancer cells from animals significantly inhibited proliferation of the cancer cells and destroyed some. As a matter of fact, the National Cancer Institute has funded much research on sulfides in onions and garlic, naming them promising agents in fending off cancer!

Potato: The potato originated in South America. Botanically, the potato is related to the eggplant. The potato is a tuber, according to Dr. Mike Samuels the author of Heart Disease. A medium potato provides only 110 calories, Vitamin C & B6, significant niacin, more potassium (don't peel, 60% is close to the skin) than a large banana, and is low in sodium. A processed potato chip has six times the calories, 400 times the fat and 250 times the salt of the same amount of a natural unprocessed potato chip. Do you think these saturated fat, sodium, and cholesterol packed potato chips might hinder you from the healthy body and longer life you deserve? If you must have your potato chips, try making your own without the great amount saturated fat, sodium, and cholesterol. Shop around for a product that can turn potato slices into fat-free, sodium-free, low-calorie potato chips.

According to Dr. John McDougall, director of the nutritional medicine clinic at St. Helena Hospital in Deer Park, California, potatoes are an excellent food for rapid weight loss (DO NOT put the fat tasty stuff on potatoes like butter, margarine, and sour cream). Potatoes are a great source of fiber and other nutrients mentioned above, help lower cholesterol while protecting against strokes and heart disease!

White raw potatoes have high concentrations of protease inhibitors, which are compounds known to void-out certain viruses and carcinogens. Of several foods, inhibitors found in the potato were found to have the strongest antiviral powers! Potato chemicals stopped viruses better than soybean inhibitors, which are considered one of the fiercest antiviral agents. Potatoes, especially the skins, are rich in chlorogenic acid, a polyphenol which prevents cell mutations leading to cancer. Potato skins were found to have antioxidant activity - neutralizing *"free radicals"* that damage cells leading to many disorders including cancer.

It's a crying shame! According to the Agriculture Department and National Cancer Institute, the closest many children get to a vegetable is eating French fries!

Sweet Potato: One medium sweet potato baked in its skin, then peeled furnishes only 160 calories. It's very nutritious, low in fat, and furnishes Vitamin A that has eight times the recommended allowance. Vitamin A in sweet potatoes comes in the form of carotene and has the potential to reduce the risk of lung cancer. The National Cancer Institute shows that eating 1/2 cup of sweet potatoes or other bright orange vegetables can reduce the likelihood of lung cancer by as much as 50 percent! Smokers have a 20-30 times higher risk of cancer than nonsmokers.

Tomatoes: A 2 1/2 inch tomato furnishes only 23 calories, provides fiber, is low in fat and sodium, and rich in vitamin A, Vitamin C, and potassium.

According to a five year study from Harvard Medical School, people that ate tomatoes or strawberries every week, had the lowest chances of dying from cancer. This fits right in with cancer-prevention recommendations that the National Cancer Institute and other groups have issued based on current knowledge of how diet affects diseases.

FRUIT

How about fruit that is healthy and tasty!

Apples: *"An Apple A Day Keeps The Doctor Away?"* The apple may be the King of the fruit world. Apples have been eaten by man since at least the New Stone Age, nearly 6,000 years ago. There are several thousand varieties of apples due to grafting; from the wild apple to produce strains that are less resistant to disease and apples that have particular flavors and colors. Two main groups of apples are sweet one's for eating and sharper varieties for cooking or making alcoholic drinks.

Apples are rich in many needed minerals and Vitamins and may help *"Keep the doctor away."* Apples are rich in soluble fiber, which has the ability to lower blood cholesterol levels and lower your blood pressure. Apples also help to dampen the appetite and the juices in apples are noted to kill infectious diseases.

According to Dr. James Anderson at the University of Kentucky School of Medicine, soluble fiber prevents hunger pangs by steadying your blood sugar level. Apples have virtually no saturated fat, cholesterol, or sodium. A medium apple furnishes only 81 calories. Apples contain pectin for those heart healthy wannabe's. Eat an apple prior to bedtime. The pectin will keep your brain chemicals levels stable throughout the night. You'll wake-up happy and refreshed!

According to studies, even the aroma of apples can also calm you down, reducing anxiety. The juices in a fresh apple are noted to be strong virus fighters.

According to a study at Michigan State University, subjects who ate two apples a day had less tension, fewer headaches, and less frequent emotional upsets.

According to a study at Yale University, researchers noted that the scent of spiced apples produced a calming effect which aids to lower blood pressure!

Bananas: A medium banana furnishes only 100 calories, has hardly any sodium, and is a modest source of Vitamin C. Bananas also furnish fiber for the heart healthy concerned and provides potassium which helps in controlling blood pressure. Bananas are also packed with Vitamin B6 which helps prevent depression. One banana provides 35% of the B6 RDA. Eating a banana helps combat hunger pangs and leaves you feeling satisfied and full. Bananas also help you remain alert and energetic because the fructose sugar that is encased in fiber and carbohydrates is slowly released into your system.

In the 1930s, medical literature noted that bananas were a cure for ulcers. Experimenting with mice, researchers isolated a chemical in ripe and unripe bananas that suppressed acid secretion, thus blocking the development of ulcers in animals.

Modern teams of British and Indian researchers have discovered why the banana-eating rodents end up with about 1/3 fewer and less severe ulcers. Bananas work just like the most sophisticated drugs (carbenoxolone), but without the side-effects like high blood pressure. Bananas strengthen the surface cells of the stomach lining, forming a sturdier barrier against noxious juices. The British researchers' bottom line: *"The role of bananas in folk medicine as an antiulcerogenic agent, at least against gastric ulcers, appears justified...."*

Berries: If you're watching your weight, try eating some berries. Berries are low calorie - low fat sweets, that have hardly any sodium, a great source of potassium, and supplies fiber that helps you absorb fewer of the calories that you do eat. Berries are also an aid in the improvement of your blood pressure. A cup of strawberries has the lowest count at only 45 calories and a cup of blueberries has the highest count of 81 calories. The calorie count for raspberries and blackberries fall in between these two very tasty treats. Berries have natural fructose sugar to satisfy your sweet-craving, therefore an aid to weight-loss!

Did you know blueberries are a common Swedish folk remedy for diarrhea? In Sweden, dried blueberry soup has been used by physicians to treat childhood diarrhea. According to Finn Sandberg, professor of pharmacology at Uppsala Biomedical Center in Sweden, 5 to 10 grams (1/3 of an ounce) of dried blueberries is the dosage for diarrhea.

Why do blueberries work so well against diarrhea? Blueberries contain high concentrations of compounds that KILL both bacteria and viruses! In Canadian tests, crushed blueberries destroyed nearly 100 percent of polio viruses within 24 hours, even when the blueberries were diluted 10 times!

Cherries: A cup of sweet red cherries furnishes 82 calories, whereas a cup of sour red cherries furnishes only 52 calories. Cherries may be a great diet aid. If you enjoy sweets, substitute that 300 calorie candy bar for cherries that will not only satisfy your sweet tooth but fill you up. Cherries are a good source of Vitamin A, low in sodium, a modest fiber content for your heart, and no fat.

According to a 1950 writing by Ludwig Blau, Ph.D., in the Texas Reports on Biology and Medicine, he cured his crippling gout that confined him to a wheelchair by eating 6 to 8 cherries each day! He noted that as long as he ate cherries, the gout stayed away! He also annotated that 12 others who suffered from gout also ate or drank cherry juice and they were also completely free of gout!

Prevention magazine printed Ludwig Blaus's advice and testimonials started to pour in to Prevention magazine! Many wrote and said initially consuming 15 to 20 red or black cherries a day then 10 a day after that worked to remedy their affliction with gout!

According to a study at Forsyth Dental Center, cherry juice is a potent antibacterial agent against tooth decay! They noted that black cherry juice blocked 80 percent of the enzyme activity leading to plaque formation, which is the groundwork to tooth decay.

Figs: The medicinal benefits of the figs go back to the Old Testament. However, modern research has already used figs to fight cancer and bacteria!

According to Japanese scientists at the Institute of Physical and Chemical Research at the Mitsubishi-Kasei Institute of Life Sciences in Tokyo, *"The use of the fig fruit as a traditional anticancer agent is widespread all over the world."*

Japanese scientist have isolated an anticancer chemical (benzaldehyde) in figs and used it to treat cancer patients. The Japanese scientists gave oral doses of the fig distillate to cancer patients with some success. Later they injected the fig chemical (benzaldehyde) with great results!

Fifty-five (55) percent of the patients with advanced cancer improved when injected with doses of a benzaldehyde derivative. Seven patients went into complete remission! Twenty-nine went into partial remission! Patients given the fig substance generally lived longer! Scientists have also isolated fig enzymes called ficins that help digestion. Fig juice has also been noted to kill bacteria and kill roundworms in dogs.

Oranges: A medium orange furnishes only 62 calories, has virtually no sodium and hardly any fat, and is a great way to get your Vitamin C. The U.S. Department of Agriculture found that almost every milligram of Vitamin C in oranges do survive the transition from the orange grove to frozen orange juice concentrate. Oranges lower the risk of some cancers, as well as effectively lowering blood cholesterol and fighting arterial plaque!

Papaya: Mexican Indians say that papaya has healing powers. A regular size papaya provides only 160 calories, Vitamin C, a significant source of folic acid, fiber, and very low in sodium. It is best to pick a papaya when it is just turning yellow. Papayas provide healthy digestive properties (enzyme called papain) that have a direct tonic effect on the stomach.

Peaches: A regular size peach has only 37 calories and provides Vitamins C and A. The skin of a peach can be removed very easily by boiling it just a minute or so and then dropping it in very cold water for a about a minute. Peaches are easily digestible and provide a high fiber content while promoting regularity.

Pears: Worldwide, pears are the second most important fruit crop after apples, but in the United States they rank third after apples and peaches. With 3,000 varieties in the Unites States, only a handful are commercially consumed. Six ounces of raw pears provide only 101 calories and 46 calories per half (dried). Pears provide a fair amount of Vitamin C and iron while aiding in digestion. Pears are an excellent source of roughage while being an aid in regularity.

Pineapples: Two slices of pineapple provide only 90 calories, Vitamin C, and very little sodium. When picking fresh pineapples at the supermarket, ensure the leaves are dark green. A natural enzyme found in pineapples, called bromelain, is a nutrient that increases the body's ability to break down fats and protein promoting body metabolism! Pineapple is rich in manganese and helps satisfy your sweet tooth!

SEAFOOD\MEAT

How about eating seafood\meat that is healthy and tasty! If you really like seafood, fish and poultry, then see U.S. Food & Drug Administration Seafood Hotline in Section 25.

Shellfish: Shellfish are low in fat, furnish fewer calories than beef, furnish a source of calcium, and are extremely tasty. Here are the calorie counts for four ounces of six types of shellfish. Shelled clams furnish only 86 calories.

Cooked crab furnishes only 105 calories. A cooked lobster furnishes only 108 calories. Canned mussels furnish only 107 calories. Shelled oysters furnish only 103 calories. Cooked scallops furnish only 127 calories.

It was once thought that shellfish were hazardous to your cardiovascular system because they elevated blood cholesterol. Well it is just the opposite. Shellfish help protect arteries and blood vessels by significantly lowering bad-type blood cholesterol (LDL). Shellfish carry high concentrations of Omega-3 fatty acids that help prevent blood clots (thrombi) in blood vessels and are noted to be potentially beneficial to many diseases including allergies, asthma, cancer, headaches, psoriasis, and rheumatoid arthritis!

Are shellfish a brain food? Shellfish, as well as other seafood, do stimulate mental energy! According to Dr. Judith Wurtman, a leading researcher at MIT, shellfish and fish boost your mood and mental performance. Why? Shellfish are low in fat and carbohydrates and almost pure protein which delivers large amounts of an amino acid called tyrosine to the brain.

Fish: Heart-health experts have found the benefits of eating fish are even greater than previously realized. In 1985 the New England Journal of Medicine found that *"the consumption of as little as one or two fish dishes per week may be of preventive importance in relation to coronary heart disease."* Omega-3 fats in fish benefits the heart by making the blood less prone to the abnormal clotting process that can lead to a heart attack.

Fresh fish rates high for keeping blood pressure in a healthy range. Jichi Medical School in Japan have shown that levels of "good" HDL cholesterol were high among Japanese who eat the most fish! Fish may also help those who suffer from arthritis.

According to Dr. Joel Kremer of Albany Medical College in New York, daily supplements of EPA (eicosapentaenoic acid) fish oil brought dramatic relief to inflammation and stiff joints caused by rheumatoid arthritis. Fish is less fattening and more digestible than beef. Fish is high in mineral selenium which has proven to chase away the blues.

Is fish a brain food? It sure is! Fish is noted to be food for thought! According to Dr. Judith Wurtman, principal investigator at MIT, the high protein in fish, namely the amino acid tyrosine, may boost the brain neurotransmitters norepinephrine and dopamine, which energizes your mind and makes you feel more alert. Three or four ounces of fish (broiled or grilled) is sufficient.

WARNING: Fast food fish is noted to have 1/10 of Omega-3 fish oil compared to a can of Chinook salmon. Fast food fish is mostly made from whitefish already low in fat and Omega-3's.
Too much Omega-3 may block normal blood clotting and lead to excessive bleeding.
Researchers have discovered that Omega-3 fish oil capsules can actually aggravate diabetes by producing a steep rise in blood sugar and a drop in insulin secretion.

Chicken: Eat chicken instead of high fat and high cholesterol red meat. Four ounces of cooked white meat provide only 245 calories, while dark meat provides 285 calories. Chicken has far less fat and cholesterol than a T-bone steak, but is equal in protein. Cook with the skin on the chicken but DO NOT EAT THE SKIN.

WARNING: Chickens are a great money-maker. To ensure those pecking chickens grow as fast as possible, some chicken farms may introduce chemicals to the chickens so they weigh the most in the least amount of time.

These chemicals are passed on to the consumer - YOU! Before you purchase that poultry, investigate where and how it was raised. You might be better off buying your chicken meat from a small poultry farmer who has no need to pump his chickens up with hormones and chemicals! You'll probably save some money too!

Turkey: A protein-rich food that elevates the brain's levels of dopamine and norepinephrine, (two neurotransmitters that help us to react quickly feel motivated, and mentally energetic). Just 04 ounces of raw turkey provides only 145 calories and only 5 grams of fat. Compare this to an equal portion of ground beef that will provide a whopping 313 calories and 23 grams of fat. Replace that ground beef with turkey; like hamburger, meat loaf, or spaghetti sauce. Eating turkey will help lower your serum cholesterol.

Veal: Veal is the leanest form of beef. It is a bit more expensive, but it provides the taste without the fat and is loaded with protein, niacin, and iron. Four ounces of cooked veal has only 244 calories.

Keys to CUTTING FAT & CALORIES IN COOKING

* Trim fat before cooking.
* Roast or broil meat on a rack.
* Brown meat, then drain fat before continuing to cook in pan.
* Remove fat (skim from top) from stews or soups after chilling.
* Use low fat cooking methods such as bake, broil, microwave, roast, stir-fry, or braise.

OTHER HEALTHY FOOD ITEMS

The following are other healthy foods you should consider consuming instead of fat-rich, sugar-rich, sodium-rich, and cholesterol-packed unhealthy foods.

Bread: Whole grain bread provides approximately 70 calories per slice. Bread is a natural source of fiber and complex carbohydrates and provides protein. Bread itself isn't fattening, it's the butter, cream cheese, margarine, and mayonnaise that you put on it. Bread can be an aid to weight-loss! According to Dr. Bjarne Jacobsen, a Norwegian scientist, people that ate less than two slices of bread on a daily basis weighed 11 pounds more than big bread eaters. According to researchers at Michigan State University, some breads actually reduce your appetite! Students who ate 12 slices of dark, high-fiber bread (pumpernickel, whole wheat, mixed grain, or oatmeal) lost five pounds in two months compared to students who ate white bread who were hungrier, ate more fattening foods and lost no weight!

WARNING: It is noted that one fake food is white flour. Approximately 98% of bread, pancakes, pastries, and spaghetti are made with white flour. Some of these products are caramel colored to make you think you are eating 100% whole wheat products. READ the ingredients or make your own bread, pancakes, and pasta. READ the important data below!

According to a special report from Vita-Mix, compared to whole wheat, white bread is missing:

* 72% of chromium   * 78% of Vitamin B-6
* 78% of dietary fiber   * 96% of Vitamin E
* 50% of folic acid   * 62% of Zinc
* 72% of magnesium   * many phytochemicals

The missing nutrients in white bread are critical to:
* appetite control
* cell communication
* fetal brain development
* immune function
* preventing free radicals
* and 500 other body functions

See Vita-Mix in Section 25.

Chili Peppers: One-half cup of chili peppers provides only 30 calories. They are rich in Vitamin A, Vitamin C, high in fiber, fat free, low in sodium, and a great source of calcium, iron, phosphorus, and magnesium. Capsaicin, the fire-causing substance in chili peppers, has been noted to lower cholesterol and triglyceride levels. Chili peppers may be a great aid to weight-loss.

According to researchers at Oxford Polytechnic Institute, adding three grams of hot chili sauce plus three grams of ordinary yellow mustard to a meal can raise a person's metabolic rate by as much as 25%! You don't have to do anything; your body will burn extra calories on its own!

Cottage Cheese: One-half cup of cottage cheese provides approximately 84 to 120 calories depending on the brand you purchase. Ensure that you purchase cottage cheese that is 1 to 2 percent milk fat. Cottage cheese provides a healthy source of calcium, Vitamin B, riboflavin, and is a great weight-loss food. Try whipping cottage cheese instead of using cream cheese. Use cottage cheese for all sorts of recipes instead of sour cream or cream cheese.

Herbs: For more years than there are words in this book, mankind has turned to herbs as a source of healing power. Herbs are from non-poisonous plants like bark, fruits, leaves, and vegetables. Animals instinctively use herbs to remedy their sickness.

Nowadays, herbs are being used by millions of people as an alternative, preventive medicine, and as their primary health care instead of conventional medicines and treatments. Herbs have a long history of success without the harmful side-effects of modern medicine and treatments. Herbs can help the body heal itself without building up residual effects or toxic side-effects. READ much more about those AMAZING herbs in Section 19.

Honey: Greeks regarded it as *"food fit for the gods!"* Besides being extremely tasty, honey is noted to be easy on the digestive system because the bees have already digested it. It acts as an antiseptic and helps relieve burns, skin abrasions, and even bee stings! Honey provides many nutrients like calcium, copper, iron, manganese, magnesium, phosphorus, potassium, silica, sodium, and Vitamin C from pollen. AVOID honey in your local grocery store, because it is heat treated and filtered. Purchase honey at health food stores. Ensure it is pure, untreated and unfiltered honey (cloudy with healthful pollen). Your best bet is to go out in the countryside and look for honey farmers. ENSURE you ask them if pesticides are used on any part of their land or neighboring farm lands. If so, the pesticides may be passed on to the honey.

Kelp: It is noted that Japanese eat great quantities of seaweed. Epidemiologists have noted that Japanese women have a fraction of breast cancer in comparison to American women. Japanese women who are diagnosed with breast cancer live longer than American and British women.

A 1974 Japanese study noted that kelp not only helps prevent the development of breast cancer, but that it could also treat existing tumors! Kelp was instrumental in slowing the progression of breast malignancies in 95% of test animals. Sixty percent of these test animals went into complete remission!

Olive Oil: Olive oil varies in quality. The term *"virgin"* is loosely applied. Originally it meant that the oil was from the first pressing of the fruit, as opposed to the second or third pressing. Olive oil when unrefined has a greenish tinge and a pungent flavor. It is preferred to refined oils because the health qualities are intact. I've found that Extra Virgin Italian Olive Oil (cold pressed), is one of the best bets for a quality oil.

Many studies have shown that populations using large amounts of olive oil like Italy and Greece have lower heart disease and stroke. Olive oil is rich in Vitamin E and a known antioxidant. Olive oil is linked to longevity, olive trees have been known to live as long as 3,000 years!

Olive oil may be one of the best choices when cooking with oils. Olive oil IS NOT saturated fat but is a monounsaturated fatty acid, which is stable at high temperatures and less prone to oxidation than other vegetable oils. Extra Virgin Oil is probably your best choice of all the other oils. Avoid refined vegetable oils.

All cooking oils are 100% fat. Vegetable oils contain a combination of saturated, monounsaturated and polyunsaturated fats in varying proportions. There is no such thing as a saturated-fat-free oil or one containing purely monounsaturated or polyunsaturated fat.

One study may contradict another study concerning the health benefits or negative results of one oil or another. One fact is agreed upon by most studies. Consuming products that have saturated fat has been linked to a very long list of diseases. The bottom line is to cut the fat. If oils are required for cooking, cook with monounsaturated fats since studies are still finding their beneficial affects towards health for you above polyunsaturated fats.

People in the Mediterranean have been noted to develop far less heart disease than Americans, even though they drink, smoke, and even consume as much or more saturated fat than Americans! What are they doing different? Their diet consists of an oil they use on their vegetables, grain-rich dishes, and meats. They even dip their bread in it! It's olive oil! Yes olive oil.

One added bonus of monounsaturated fats is they maintain HDL (high density lipoprotein) that helps prevent heart disease. Olive, peanut and canola oils are noted to be highest in monounsaturated fats. Ensure you read the Nutrition Facts label on any cooking oil. Look for the word *"monounsaturated."* Look for the least amount of saturated fats and the most monounsaturated fats.

WARNING: ENSURE you use *"cold pressed"* olive oil! Use all cooking oils sparingly! Read about cholesterol in Section 08.

Why are people who live by the Mediterranean Diet, healthier than Americans despite their high tobacco consumption, low exercise level, and modest health-care system?

The Mediterranean Diet is a diet low in meat, but high in cereal, fruit, grain, legumes, monounsaturated fats, nuts, and vegetables. Recent French Study found that the Mediterranean Diet after a heart attack was 70 percent more life-saving than the Standard American Diet (low-fat diet-less than 30 percent fat calories). Some Harvard Researchers favor the Mediterranean Diet over the Standard American Diet.

A research effort called the Seven Countries Study, examined 12,763 men ages 40 through 59 in the Netherlands, Finland, Italy, Greece, Croatia and Serbia, Japan, and the United States. Ten years after their initial screening, the study reported several important results:

- Mediterranean groups had lower death rates from all causes than   the northern European and American groups.

- Lower mortality from coronary heart disease in the Mediterranean countries.

- Men at the peak of their lives (45 years) have longer life expectancies in Greece than in any other European or North American country despite their high tobacco consumption, low exercise level, and modest health-care system.

Pasta: Pasta is found in many cuisines throughout the world like Italian lasagna, Chinese lo mein, Greek pistachio, and Jewish lokshen kugel. Did you know pasta isn't fattening? Pasta itself provides approximately 110 calories per ounce, but the fattening stuff is what you add to the pasta (butter, cheese, oil, tomato sauce, and ground beef.)! Pasta is rich in copper, iron, magnesium, manganese, niacin, phosphorus, protein, riboflavin, thiamin, and zinc. Pasta is easily digestible, low in fat, and low in sodium. Eat some pasta but watch what you put on it!

Rice: Rice is not only delicious, but filling and good for you. Rice contains only a trace of fat, a source of complex carbohydrates, is cholesterol free, and has approximately 164 calories per cup. Brown rice still has the outer kernel or outer covering which makes brown rice higher in fiber and nutrients than white rice.

In the one study, Dr. Walter Kempner at Duke University, Durham, North Carolina, developed the Rice Diet. Rice was the staple food; fruits and then vegetables were later added to the diet. The Rice Diet produced weight-loss, reversed and cured kidney ailments, as well as helped remedy high blood pressure! If you desire to try the Rice Diet, read as much as you can concerning this diet and seek your physician's advice.

Skim Milk: One cup of skim milk has only a trace of fat. One cup of 2-percent-fat milk has 5 grams of fat, while 1 cup of whole milk has 8 grams of fat.

ANTI-FAT FOODS AND SPICES

According to Isabelle Martin, author of Foods That Make You Lose Weight or Negative Calories, the following foods can be labeled as ANTI-FAT FOODS because they burn as many calories as they supply. These foods contain 75 to 95 percent water and an average of 25 calories an ounce. So what are you waiting for, eat up!!!

Spices stimulate the digestive juices and contribute to the to the DESTRUCTION OF FAT. Hot Mustard in particular can temporarily speed up the metabolism as much as 7 to 8 hours. Research has indicated that the metabolic rates goes up ten (10) percent after a meal. This is called the *"thermic effect."*

The lower the fat content the higher the *"thermic effect."* This *"thermic effect"* can double if you do some light exercise one-half hour after you've eaten. A study conducted at Stanford University showed that light exercise burns 2000 calories per week, speeds up weight loss and is good for your heart.

ANTI-FAT FOODS: Artichoke, Asparagus, Beets, Broccoli, Cauliflower, Celery, Chicory, Cucumber, Dandelion, Endives, Green Beans, Green peppers, Green Cabbage, Horseradish, Lettuce, Onion, Radish, Spinach, Swiss Chard, Turnip, Watercress, and Zucchini.

As a matter of fact, most of the fruits and vegetables in EAT THE RIGHT STUFF may be considered FAT-FIGHTING FOODS, as long as your diet is low in fat and consist of the foods that are listed above. The vegetables and fruits in this section are all very low in fat content and provide a deluge of other health benefits for you now and are a good healthy investment for your future. A healthy diet, drinking good, clean, contaminant-free water, and exercise go hand-in-hand.

WARNING: SEE YOUR DOCTOR prior to any dieting or exercise plan.

ANTI-FAT SPICES: Basil, Clove, Fennel, Garlic, Mint, Parsley, Sage, Savory, Tarragon, and Thyme.

FIVE FOOD GROUPS

Dietary Guidelines for Americans

What should Americans eat to stay healthy?
The Standard American Diet has too many calories, too much fat, too much cholesterol, and too much sodium. The American diet has too little complex carbohydrates and fiber. Such a diet is linked to America's high rates of obesity and of certain diseases: heart disease, high blood pressure, stroke, diabetes, and some forms of cancer. Food alone cannot make you absolutely 100% healthy. Good health also depends on your heredity, your environment, and the health care you get. Your lifestyle is very important: how much do you exercise, do you smoke, are you around second-hand smoke, do you abuse alcohol, do you abuse drugs.

The first guideline for eating to stay healthy is EAT A VARIETY OF FOODS. The second guideline is to CHANGE YOUR DIET TO BE LOWER IN SATURATED FAT, HIGHER IN COMPLEX CARBOHYDRATES & FIBER. The third guideline is MODERATE USE OF SUGARS, SALT, and if used at all alcoholic beverages and tobacco products.

You need more than 40 different nutrients for good health. Essential nutrients include Vitamins, minerals, amino acids from protein, certain fatty acids from fat and sources of calories (protein, carbohydrates, and fat). One way to assure variety is to choose foods each day from five major food groups. Individuals who do not eat foods from one or more of the food groups may want to contact a dietitian for help in planning how to meet nutritional needs.

FIVE FOOD GROUPS	SUGGESTED SERVINGS
Vegetables	03 to 05 servings
Fruits	02 to 04 servings
Breads, Cereals, Rice & Pasta	06 to 11 servings
Milk, Yogurt & Cheese	02 to 03 servings
Meats, Poultry, Fish, Dry Beans and Peas, Eggs and Nuts.	02 to 03 servings

Consume saturated fats, hydrogenated oils, refined sugars, and sodium SPARINGLY (avoid completely if possible).

Choose a Diet Low in Cholesterol, Saturated Fat, Sodium, and Sugar.

Most health authorities recommend a diet with less saturated fat and cholesterol. Populations like the American populace, which have diets high in fat, have higher percentages of obesity and certain types of cancer. Diets that have higher levels of saturated fat and cholesterol are linked to increased risk for heart disease.

A diet low in saturated fat and cholesterol may help to maintain a desirable level of blood cholesterol. For adults, this level is below 200 mg/dl. As blood cholesterol increases above this level, greater risk for heart disease occurs. Heart disease risk may increase by high blood pressure, cigarette smoking, diabetes, history of heart disease in the family, obesity, and being male.

Table salt contains sodium and chloride. Both sodium and chloride are essential in the diet. However, most Americans eat far too much salt. Many foods already contain the sodium needed in our diet. In the U.S, one in three adults has high blood pressure. If these people restrict their salt and sodium, usually their blood pressure will fall. It is important for most people eat less salt and sodium. Reduction will benefit those people with high blood pressure as well as a preventative for those who haven't high blood pressure.

Americans eat sugars in many forms. Both sugars and starches, which break down into sugars, can contribute to tooth decay. Sugars and starches are in many foods that also supply nutrients-milk, fruits, some vegetables, breads, cereals, and other foods.

If You Have To Drink Alcoholic Beverages, Do So in Moderation. Alcoholic beverages supply calories but little or no nutrients. Drinking them has no health benefit, is linked with many health problems, is the cause of many accidents, and can lead to addiction. Women who are pregnant or trying to conceive should AVOID consuming alcohol. Major birth defects have been attributed to heavy drinking by the mother while pregnant. There is no conclusive evidence that an occasional drink is harmful, but why take a chance and make a mistake that will last you and your baby a lifetime!

Individuals who plan on driving or engaging in other activities that require attention or skill should REFRAIN from consuming alcohol. Most people retain some alcohol in the blood 3 to 5 hours after even moderate drinking.

What's moderate drinking?
Women: No more than 01 drink a day.
Men: No more than 02 drinks a day.
A drink: 12 ounces of regular beer or 05 ounces of wine or 1 1/2 ounces of distilled spirits (80 proof).

SECTION 02 - THE GOOD THE BAD AND THE UGLY

The following is very important healthy information. Once you read this section along with the others, you'll soon realize how all this information is interrelated towards a healthier you once you take the proper action. Avoid and fight heart disease, cancer, stroke, and a multitude of other diseases! So please read on.

The Good -- Fiber: Fiber comes from plant foods. There is no fiber in foods like eggs, beef, cheese, chicken, or pork. Fiber is not digested; it provides no calories. Fiber speeds up the elimination of waste and combats constipation. Fiber helps remove cholesterol (lowers cholesterol) and cancer-causing chemicals out of your bodies system. Nutritionists recommend at least 35 grams and up to 70 grams of daily fiber. Fiber helps food pass through the intestines faster and lowers the absorption of fat! So if you eat any fatty foods ensure that fiber is consumed during your meal. A diet high in fiber can be a factor in lowering cholesterol levels. Remember, fiber comes from plant foods. Read the Nutritional Facts on all food products that you purchase. Stay away from the foods that are high in saturated fats, sodium and cholesterol. Choose foods that are have little or no fats, sodium and cholesterol but have ample protein, carbohydrates, fiber, and Vitamins.

The Good -- Antioxidants: Antioxidants absorb free radicals by making them complete which in turn make them harmless. Some good antioxidants are selenium, zinc, Vitamins A, C, and E. Read about Free Radicals and Antioxidants in Section 09.

The Bad -- Free Radicals: A free radical is an atom or group of atoms that has at least one unpaired electron. Because another element can easily pick up this free electron and cause a chemical reaction, these free radicals can effect dramatic and destructive changes in the body. Read the section on Free Radicals and Antioxidants in Section 09.

HOW MUCH FAT IS IN THE FOOD? DO THE MATH!

Use this formula to determine HOW MUCH FAT a product contains, before you buy it.

Step 1 -- Multiply 09 (number of calories per gram of fat) by the number of fat grams per serving stated on the label.

Step 2 -- Divide this number of total fat calories by the number of total calories per serving.

Step 3 -- Multiply your answer by 100.

Example: 09 times 04 (calories per gram of fat) = 36.

36 divided by 200 (total calories per serving) = .18

.18 times 100 = 18.

This package is 18% calories from fat (noodle soup).

The Bad -- Cholesterol: Cholesterol's job is to carry fat through your blood vessels. Fat cannot travel through your blood vessels on it's own because fat doesn't mix with water and water is a major ingredient in blood. Cholesterol does this very well and in a healthy way until there is too much fat content in your diet along with Bad Cholesterol.

The Ugly -- Blood Pressure (High): Nearly 60 million Americans have high blood pressure or hypertension. When cholesterol build-up causes arteries to narrow, your heart pumps harder to push the blood through your arteries. Pressure on your arteries walls is stronger and High Blood Pressure\Hypertension is the result. Hypertension is a life threatening disease.

SECTION 03 - EXERCISE AND THE RIGHT DIET, IT'S NEVER TOO LATE TO FEEL GOOD AGAIN

According to Webster's New World Medical Dictionary exercise is: Bodily exertion for the sake of restoring the organs and functions to a healthy state or keeping them healthy.

According to researchers at Scripps College, exercise keeps your brain in shape. Research indicates that there is a 20% difference in the ability to reason & remember and physical reaction times between people who exercise and couch potatoes.

Benefits from regular exercise are improved self-confidence, increased capacity for physical work, increased endurance, increased muscle tone, reduced risk of heart attack, and weight loss\control.

Do Diets Work?
If you don't know it by now, dieting is a mega big bucks business. Most of those companies that promote their weight-loss programs do not keep accurate information on their results. Informal surveys have demonstrated that VERY FEW dieters will have maintained their weight-loss 12 months later. Who benefits from these diets? Probably the person selling those diet programs.

Is there a weight-loss program that does work?
Many studies have noted that healthy eating habits, meaning EAT THE RIGHT STUFF, STARTING AND MAINTAINING AN EXERCISE PROGRAM and losing weight gradually are the most effective ways of reducing your weight PERMANENTLY! Replace fat with complex carbohydrates and protein. Supplements of Vitamins and minerals are also recommended.

When I exercise, should I go for the gold or exercise at a rate to just break a sweat?
First of all, ensure you see your doctor prior to implementing any exercise program or diet. As far as exercise, stay within your ability as per your doctor's instructions and EAT THE RIGHT STUFF!

According to a study at the Cooper Institute for Aerobic Research in Dallas, overweight women were divided into three groups of fast walkers, moderate walkers, and the slowpokes. Guess who lost the most fat? The slowpokes! Why? According to Dr. John Duncan, it's theorized that the body burns two types of fuel - glycogen which we'll say is high-octane fuel and the other fuel is fat which we'll call low-octane. If you're really going fast, you're going to use high-octane fuel (glycogen), whereas if you're taking it easy, your using low-octane fuel (fat)!

The following ARE NOT EXCUSES for lack of exercise!
- I don't have the time.
- I'm too tired to exercise.
- I'm too out of shape. I'm too far gone.
- I'm too old.
- I'm disabled.

ACTIVITIES THAT BURN CALORIES

Exercise is the active use of the body to build or maintain strength, endurance, to make the body healthier, and it burns calories! A 170 pound person can burn 95 calories per hour just sitting (110-pound person burns 65 calories), whereas the same 170 pound person can burn as much as 600 calories per hour running a 10 minute mile (110 lb person burns 360 calories). The following are common activities of one hour duration and the calories burnt for a 170 pound person. Use your best judgment (or purchase a Calorie Burner Scale from any grocery store) to determine the calories burnt calories.

Activity	Calories Burnt
Slow Dancing	235
Fast Dancing	475
Fishing	290
Mowing the lawn	515
Golfing	390

Activity	Calories Burnt
Ironing	150
Mopping	285
Shopping	285
Swimming Slow	595
Swimming Fast	720
Tennis	505
Typing	125
Volleyball (6 people)	295
Walking	360
Weight Training	850

What about all those exercise machines - should I buy one to get in shape?

First of all, ensure you see your doctor prior to implementing any new exercise program. Second see a fitness expert and relate your fitness goals. The fitness expert could guide you in the right direction whether it be weight training, cardiovascular type workouts and the list goes on.

If you do decide to purchase any type of exercise machine ENSURE you try it out and ensure you feel comfortable with it and YOU WILL USE ON A REGULAR BASIS! Some machines like the cross-country skiing machine may take a day or so to learn but it's noted to be an excellent workout!

Below are some tips and general information on various exercise machines and exercises.

Cross-Country Skiing: Cross-Country skiing machines actually work most muscles. The legs are used to shuffle the skis forward and back while the arms and upper-body muscles push and mostly pull the simulated poles. The top-of-the-line machines, leg and upper body resistance can be increased as well as the incline. Computers that monitor time, speed, and heart rate are available. Because of its success and popularity, cross-country ski machines are manufactured by many companies making a wide variety of different models. Look at most health related magazines and you'll see one company called NordicTrack. I (author) purchased a NordicTrack Achiever and have had many a great workouts on it!

Rower: Rowing machines are noted to work all major muscle groups (abdominals, arms, back, buttocks and legs). Rowing is non-impact as compared to running, and dance aerobics. An aerobic exercise as well as providing strength conditioning (upper and lower body), rowing burns calories faster than biking (level of exertion is the same). Rowing also enhances flexibility because of the wider range of motion of pushing, pulling, and bending.

The American college of Sports Medicine recommends rowing because it is the single exercise which best develops the combination of flexibility, strength, and cardiovascular fitness!

Stair Climber: Stair climbing firms and tones the legs and buttocks, and improves running performance. A low-impact exercise, it's non-jarring climbing motion won't harm joints. Stair Climber machines build strength, endurance, and aerobic conditioning in one exercise! Your workout results will be different and more challenging depending on the type of stair climber machine you utilize. Most regular standard type stair climber machines utilize the larger muscles of the body (leg muscles) and with consistent workouts, you should see results soon!

Water Exercise: How would you like a good workout without the unnecessary wear and tear on your joints and muscles? It's called water exercise! Water exercise provides 12 times the resistance in water compared to the same exercise in air (outside the pool) and WITHOUT the unnecessary wear and tear on your joints and muscles! It's a great cardiovascular workout and a great upper and lower body workout! If you want extra resistance, water noodles, water paddles, and water balls will definitely add that extra challenge! Water exercise is noted to be beneficial for pregnant women and those suffering from arthritis. Arthritis sufferers may want to conduct water exercises in a facility that provides much warmer water temperatures and a special staff! Look in your local telephone directory and start calling today for the right facility and schedule for YOU!

EXERCISE EQUIPMENT POINTS OF CONTACT LIST

Besides a healthy diet, exercise is one of best ways to get healthy and stay that way! ENSURE you consult with your doctor prior to initiating any exercise program. Below are multiple Points of Contact that provide health-enhancing exercise machines and equipment. These are the BEST companies in the U.S. and the world! With the proper diet, the correct supplements, and the right exercise machine(s) - along with a good training schedule:
* A couch potato can turn into a healthy looking and energetic person.
* A healthy looking and energetic person can turn into a challenging athlete.
* An athlete (amateur or professional) into a potential World Class Athlete!

Call all these companies Monday through Friday during regular business hours and request free information! THE NUMBERS BELOW ARE NOT UPDATED.

Abdominal Machines
* AB Shaper------------------------------------1-800-595-9452
* AB Works (NordicTrack)------------------1-800-851-8158*
* Total Gym-------------------------------------1-800-308-5800*

Cross Country Ski Machines
* Fitness Master---------------------------------1-800-328-8995
* NordicTrack------------------------------------1-800-328-5888*
* Precor---1-800-477-3267
* Quinton Fitness Equipment------------------1-800-426-0337*

Rider Machines
* CTX (NordicTrack)----------------------------1-800-445-2606*
* HealthRider-------------------------------------1-800-806-3651
* NordicRider Plus (NordicTrack)-------------1-800-445-2606*
* ProForm--1-800-517-4554

Rowing Machines
* Concept II--------------------------------------1-800-245-5676*
* Total Gym---------------------------------------1-800-308-5800*
* Tunturi--1-800-827-8717*
* WaterRower Inc.--------------------------------1-800-852-2210*

Stair Climbers
* Life Fitness-------------------------------------1-800-735-3867*
* NordicTrack-------------------------------------1-800-445-2606*
* Precor--1-800-477-3267
* Quinton Fitness Equipment----------------------1-800-426-0337*
* StairMaster Sports\Medical Products-----------1-800-635-2936*
* Trotter--1-800-677-6544*
* Tunturi---1-800-827-8717*

Stationary Bicycles
* Cybex---1-800-645-5392*
* Life Fitness--1-800-735-3867
* NordicTrack---1-800-445-2606*
* Precor---1-800-477-3267
* Quinton Instrument Company)--------------------1-800-426-0337*
* Tunturi--1-800-827-8717*

Strength Training Equipment
* Bowflex---1-800-BOWFLEX*
* Lifeline International Inc.----------------------------1-800-553-6633*
* NordicTrack---1-800-445-2360*
* Paramount Fitness Equipment----------------------1-800-421-6242*
* Total Gym--1-800-308-5800*
* Trotter---1-800-677-6544*
* Universal Gym Equipment--------------------------1-800-843-3906

Treadmills
Life Fitness--1-800-735-3867
NordicTrack---1-800-445-2606*
Precor---1-800-477-3267
Trotter---1-800-677-6544*
Tunturi--1-800-827-8717*
Universal Gym Equipment---------------------------1-800-843-3906

* = SEE Section 25 for more FREE information!

SECTION 04 - Cardiovascular Disease,1st Leading Killer Of Americans!

What is the heart and what does it do?

The heart is a constant working muscle that beats approximately 100,000 times and pumps 4,000 gallons of blood each 24 hours! The amazing work your heart does in one single day is equal to lifting 100 pounds one foot off the ground 1,500 times! In your lifetime, your heart will pump some 400,000 tons of blood without rest! Amazing isn't it! The heart provides life required nutrients and oxygen to all tissues of the body and even the heart itself.

What is heart disease?

The heart has a separate circulatory system which nourishes the heart with nutrients and oxygen. This circulatory system is made-up of two coronary arteries that are about the size of a pencil. These two coronary arteries subdivide and encircle the entire heart. Heart disease is the result of atherosclerosis. Atherosclerosis sometimes called *"hardening of the arteries."* It's a progressive condition in which deposits of cholesterol and lipids and other cellular waste accumulate on the inner walls of coronary arteries. This accumulation of cholesterol, lipids, and cellular waste becomes plaque. As the plaque accumulates, blood vessels become inelastic and clogged. This leads to arteries that harden and become clogged. At times, a blood clot will form on the plaque buildup and block the entire artery. A heart attack or stroke is imminent. Basically cardiovascular disease takes the form in one or more of the following manners:

- Plaque that narrows arteries, inhibiting blood flow.
- Accumulation of sticky fragments, called platelets, that form clots.
- Spasms of arteries and blood vessels, creating restrictions that stop the heart and shut-off the blood to the brain - causing strokes.

Did you know every 02 minutes one woman dies of heart disease. Approximately 40 million Americans suffer from heart disease alone! Far too many will die because they were diagnosed too late, follow an unhealthy diet, and are ignorant of many healthy alternatives to recovery.

Cardiovascular disease (commonly called heart disease) is the #1 KILLER of Americans killing approximately 500,387 women and 457,211 men each year (1993 data from the American Heart Association)! If conventional and alternative medicines could find a healthy blend of treatments, multitudes of patients afflicted with heart disease and many other diseases and maladies would be spared.

What is a heart attack?

A heart attack (myocardial infarction) occurs when one or more of the coronary arteries is partially blocked by atherosclerosis and a blood clot plugs the remaining opening. The part of the heart muscle beyond the blockage is deprived of oxygen which results in injury or death of that part of the heart muscle. If that part of the heart muscle is large enough or is a vital area of the heart, the casualty will die. Heart disease is the number one cause of death and disability in the United States. In 1988, it was estimated $60 billion was spent on the treatment and care of heart attack victims (hospitalization, loss of work, medication, and therapies).

What are some warning signs of an impending heart attack?
- Pressure, fullness, squeezing pain in the center of the chest lasting 02 minutes or more.
- Pain spreading to the shoulders, neck, jaw, arms, or back.
- Severe pain, lightheadedness, fainting, sweating, nausea and/or shortness of breath.

WARNING: All signs may not occur in every heart attack. If one symptom occurs get help immediately. Warning signs may even be different between men and women. See your doctor.

Are there any other tips I should know to guard against heart disease?

Richard Passwater, Ph.D., author of Supernutrition for Healthy Hearts offers his Total Protection Plan:
- A for Antioxidant Nutrients
- B for Blood Pressure
- C for Cigarettes (Quit or at least Reduce)
- D for Diet
- E for Exercise
- F for Fun (not Frustration)

You should seriously consider a *"Heart Check-up."* Some hospitals periodically offer this service for a nominal fee or see your doctor. The basic *"heart check-up"* should include:
- Complete lipid profile total blood cholesterol, LDL and HDL cholesterol, triglyceride level, and a coronary risk assessment. (A 12-hour fasting prior to this test is required to attain accurate readings).

43

- Diabetes Test
- Blood Pressure Test
- Height and Weight
- Baseline EKG

Are you at Risk for Heart Disease?

Take this heart disease test. If you check any of these items SEE your physician as soon as possible.

___ Bad eating habits\habits (saturated fats, cholesterol, sugar, salt, no fiber, no fruits, no vegetables, drinks alcohol, smokes). If you can't answer some of these questions you need an immediate check-up (physical)!

___ Diabetes

___ Family history of cardiovascular disease

___ High Total Cholesterol Level

___ Low HDL level (good cholesterol)

___ High LDL level (bad cholesterol)

___ High Triglycerides

___ Hypertension (high blood pressure)

___ Male

___ Overweight

___ Personal history of cardiovascular disease

___ Physical inactivity

___ Post-menopausal female

SECTION 05 - CANCER, 2ND LEADING KILLER OF AMERICANS

What is cancer?

Cancer is a group of more than 100 different diseases. Cancer occurs when cells become abnormal and keep dividing and forming more cells without control and order. All organs of the body are made up of cells. Normally, cells divide to produce more cells only when the body needs them. This order process helps keep us healthy. If cells keep dividing when new cells are not needed, a mass of tissue forms. This mass of tissue, called a growth or tumor, can be benign or malignant. Each year there are approximately 500,000 cancer deaths! That's 500,000 Americans each year! That's more than 1,300 lives EACH AND EVERY DAY OF THE YEAR! As a matter of fact there were 550,000 cancer deaths in 1995! An estimated 1,250,000 new cases of cancer for 1996 and 6 out of 10 cancer victims won't survive 5 years! These are figures for the United States alone! Think of the total world cancer deaths alone, not to mention the total deaths from heart disease, infectious diseases, stroke, diabetes, and degenerative diseases.

The American Cancer Society funds lifesaving cancer research, prevention and detection programs to effectively deal with a cancer diagnosis. To date, the American Cancer Society has invested more than $1.5 billion in lifesaving cancer research and overall more than $100 billion has been spent on finding a cure for cancer from a myriad of government and private agencies!

What are some preventive cancer exams that can be done for men?

Skin - Check for sores that do not heal. Changes in the size, shape, or color of any moles or any other changes on the skin. Report these symptoms to your doctor immediately.

Colon and Rectum - Beginning at the age of 50, you should have a yearly fecal occult blood test. The fecal occult blood test checks for blood in the stool because cancer of the colon and rectum may cause bleeding. Noncancerous conditions may also cause bleeding in the rectum and colon.

Only a test at a lab or your doctor's office can make the proper diagnosis. Your doctor checks for cancer of the rectum by inserting a gloved finger into the rectum feeling for any bumps or abnormal areas. Every 03 to 05 years after the age of 50, you should have a sigmoidoscopy. During a sigmoidoscopy, your doctor uses a thin, flexible tube with a light to look inside the rectum and colon for abnormal areas.

Mouth - During a regular visit to your doctor or dentist, your mouth should be examined for cancer and lesser medical problems like cavities and such. You can give yourself an exam by checking for the following symptoms: By looking in a mirror check for changes in color of the lips, gums, tongue, or inner cheeks for scabs, cracks, sores, white patches, swelling, or bleeding. It is often possible to see or feel changes in the mouth that might be cancer or a condition that might lead to cancer. Oral exams are especially important for people who use alcohol or tobacco products and for anyone over age 50.

Prostate - Men over the age of 40 should have a yearly digital rectal exam to check the prostate gland for hard or lumpy areas. Your doctor feels the prostate through the walls of the rectum.

Testicles - Testicular cancer occurs most often between the ages of 15 to 34. Most testicular cancers are found by self-examination. If you find a lump or notice another change, such as heaviness, swelling, unusual tenderness or pain, you should see your doctor. Ensure your doctor does a testicular exam during your regular medical checkup.

Can you give me some general cancer facts for men?
Colon and Rectum Cancer: There are more than 75,000 new cases of colon and rectum cancer diagnosed each year. It is most likely to strike men over 50 years of age. Early detection can save 4 out of 5 men. See your doctor if you are bleeding from the rectum, blood in your stool, persistent change in your bowel movements, and cramping in your abdomen.

Prostate Cancer - Approximately 35,000 American men die each year from cancer of the prostate gland. Early detection can add 5 years of life to 9 out of 10 men. Men over 65 are most likely to get prostate cancer.

If you're over 40, have a digital exam each year. If your over 50, have a prostate-specific antigen blood test every year. See your doctor if you have a painful or burning urination, see blood in your urine, or have an inability to urinate or difficulty in starting to urinate.

Testicular Cancer - Testicular cancer is most likely to strike men between the ages of 15 to 34 years of age. Testicular cancer affects the male reproductive organs. Once a month, do a self-exam. See your doctor if you find a painless swelling, feeling of heaviness, find a lump the size of a pea and have been told that your testicles have never descended.

What are some preventive cancer exams that can be done for women?

Skin - Check for sores that do not heal. Changes in the size, shape, or color of any moles or any other changes on the skin. Report these symptoms to your doctor immediately.

Colon and Rectum - Beginning at the age of 50, you should have a yearly fecal occult blood test. The fecal occult blood test checks for blood in the stool because cancer of the colon and rectum may cause bleeding. Noncancerous conditions may also cause bleeding in the rectum and colon. Only a test at a lab or your doctor's office can make the proper diagnosis. Your doctor checks for cancer of the rectum by inserting a gloved finger into the rectum feeling for any bumps or abnormal areas. Every 3 to 5 years after the age of 50, you should have a sigmoidoscopy. During a sigmoidoscopy, your doctor uses a thin, flexible tube with a light to look inside the rectum and colon for abnormal areas.

Mouth - During a regular visit to your doctor or dentist, your mouth should be examined for cancer or lesser medical problems like a cavity. You can give yourself an exam by checking for the following symptoms: By looking in a mirror check for changes in color of the lips, gums, tongue, or inner cheeks for scabs, cracks, sores, white patches, swelling, or bleeding.

It is often possible to see or feel changes in the mouth that might be cancer or a condition that might lead to cancer. Oral exams are especially important for people who use alcohol or tobacco products and for anyone over age 50.

Breasts - When breast cancer is found early, a woman has more treatment choices and a good chance of complete recovery. It is important that breast cancer be detected as early as possible. The National Cancer Institute (NCI) encourages women to take an active part in early detection of breast cancer. Each woman should talk to their doctor about breast cancer, symptoms, and a schedule for future checkups. Each woman should ask their doctor about mammograms, breast exams, and breast self-examination (BSE). Mammograms can detect many breast cancers before a BSE. Each year approximately 182,000 American women are struck with breast cancer and approximately 42,000 lives are claimed because of it.

Cervix - Regular pelvic exams and Pap test are important to detect early cancer of the cervix. According to a panel co-chairman Dr. Allen Lichter of the University of Michigan, Ann Arbor, "... we could eradicate this form of cancer." Each year approximately 15,700 women get cervical cancer and 4,900 die from it each year. Experts recommend that pap smears are done every one to three years depending on the woman's risk factors.

However studies indicate at least a third of women don't follow the guidelines. Studies indicate regular pap smears could save 4,900 lives per year! Do the math, if regular pap smears were conducted by each woman according to her risk, how many women would die of cervical cancer?

Can you give me some general cancer facts for women?
Breast Cancer - Breast cancer is one of the leading cancer killers for women. 01 in 09 women will get it. More than 46,000 American women die each year from breast cancer. Breast cancer is more likely to happen to women who are over 50 years of age, have family members with breast cancer, never had children and were over 30 years of age when they had their first child. The good news is that nearly 09 out of 10 women could survive breast cancer.

Uterine Cancer (Cervical\Endometrial) - Approximately 44,500 new cases of uterine cancer are diagnosed each year. Uterine cancer can strike women at any age. Pap tests detect signs of cervical cancer early, usually in time to treat it. Have a Pap test done if you are over 18 years of age or if you are sexually active.

Colon and Rectum Cancer - Approximately 75,000 new cases of colon and rectum cancer are diagnosed each year. It is the third major cancer killer of women. It most often strikes women over 50 years of age. Early detection can save 4 out of 5 women.

What can I do to decrease the odds of getting cancer?
First of all, see your doctor for regular physical exams. If you smoke, QUIT. See Section 25 for many organizations that could help you quit smoking and inform you about cancer, their causes, symptoms, early detection and other related information. Stay away from secondhand smoke. Get regular check-ups from your physician and EAT THE RIGHT STUFF. Curb your diet away from SATURATED fats and watch your cholesterol intake. Eat healthy meals with plenty of fruits, vegetables, fiber and good clean water. If you must drink alcohol, curb your drinking habit.

Exercise on a regular basis and get to a healthy weight according to your build and age. Read this entire book and listen to and view all 14 audio and video cassette tapes.

Sixty percent of deaths from CANCER may be preventable!

- Don't smoke or chew tobacco (lung, throat, bladder, kidney, pancreas, and mouth cancers).
- Eat less high-fat foods, avoid obesity (colon, breast, and prostate cancers).
- Eat more high-fiber foods like fruits and vegetables (colon and many other cancers).
- Respect the sun's rays. Use sun screen with SPF 15 or higher (skin cancer).
- Limit drinking of alcohol. Heavy use of alcohol, especially if you smoke or chew tobacco, increases your risk of cancer (liver, throat, and larynx cancers).

Why is everybody coming down on smokers, demanding smoke-free areas at the work place, a smoke-free environment in public places and smoke-free public transportation?
First of all nonsmokers outnumber smokers 03 to 01. Nonsmokers aren't happy about breathing passive smoke (air polluted by tobacco smoke).

The American Heart Association (AHA) and the Environmental Protection Agency (EPA) issued the unhealthy reports of secondhand smoke. The American Heart Association reports that *"secondhand smoking causes 53,000 deaths per year (37,000 of these from heart disease)."* In 1993, the EPA officially declared *"secondhand smoke to be a human carcinogen that causes about 3,000 nonsmokers a year to die from lung cancer and about 12,000 deaths a year from other cancers."* The EPA also reported that *"children exposed to secondhand smoke are at an increased risk of bronchitis, pneumonia and asthma."*

What about carcinogenic foods?
Some foods like pickled, salted, or smoked foods, especially meats are known carcinogenic. Cured meat (looks red) has been treated with nitrate preservatives which might form carcinogenic compounds in the stomach, which increase the risk of stomach and esophageal cancer. Any food that becomes moldy, especially grains, nuts, and seeds, may put you at risk. These molds frequently produce carcinogens as metabolic by-products. Vegetables like celery, cultivated white mushrooms, and peanuts have natural carcinogenic properties and should be eaten in moderation.

Meats and other proteins become carcinogenic when they are seared black over open flames or on a charcoal grill. NEVER eat the charred meat. Cut the burned portions from the main portion. NEVER inhale the smoke of burning meat or fat. Avoid carcinogenic caused cooking methods like barbecuing, charcoal broiling, frying, grilling, and smoking.

Try less carcinogenic caused cooking like baking, boiling, microwave cooking, oven broiling, poaching, and stewing.

Are there any promising drugs to treat cancer in the near future?
According to Mace Rothenburg M.D., a researcher at the University of Texas Health Science Center in San Antonio, *"There are more exciting new anticancer drugs in development than ever before. In the next few years, they are likely to have a significant impact on how we treat some common cancers."*

Throughout the United States, many researchers are pinning their hopes on antibiotics! Besides killing disease-causing bacteria, some promising antibiotics can slow down or even stop the growth of new blood vessels that cancer tumors generate to keep themselves nourished, thus preventing tumors from growing and the cancer goes into remission. Amazing antibiotics like minocycline and TNP-470.

TYPE OF CANCER	NEW CASES (1996)	DEATHS EXPECTED
Bladder Cancer	52,900	11,700
Breast Cancer	185,700	44,560
Colorectal Cancer	94,500-colon 39,000-rectum 133,500-Total	46,400-colon 8,500-rectum 54,900-Total
Kidney Cancer	30,600	12,000
Leukemia	27,600	21,000

TYPE OF CANCER	NEW CASES (1996)	DEATHS EXPECTED
Lung Cancer	177,000	158,700
Melanoma of the Skin	38,300	7,300
Non-Hodgkin's Lymphoma	52,700	23,300
Ovarian Cancer	26,700	14,800
Pancreatic Cancer	26,300	27,800
Prostate Cancer	317,100	41,400
Uterine Cancer	15,700-cervical 34,000-endometrial 49,700-Total	4,900-cervical 6,000-endometrial 15,700-Total

Source: Published from Scientific America, Special Issue - What You Need To Know About Cancer, September 1996. See Scientific America in Section 25.

SECTION 06 - MORE LEADING KILLERS OF AMERICANS, INFECTIOUS DISEASES AND STROKE

What are infectious diseases?

An infectious disease is one caused by one or more kinds of parasites (pathogen - generator of suffering) invading a susceptible human. The pathogen only wants to eat and reproduce. The pathogen may release toxic chemicals or damage essential parts of cells or organs. There are approximately 400 diseases currently considered infectious.

What's the big deal - aren't antibiotics defeating most infectious diseases?

At one time, medical doctors predicted that the development of antibiotics would undoubtedly defeat infectious diseases. However, on January 16, 1996, medical doctors in 21 nations published 242 studies to depict the scope of the threat. The most alarming news is that the death rate from infectious diseases in the United States alone rose 58 percent between 1980 and 1992. According to the Centers for Disease Control & Prevention (CDC) in Atlanta, Georgia, in 1992, infectious diseases claimed 166,000 American lives. Stroke was the 3rd leading killer of Americans, now infectious diseases claimed its place, dropping stroke to 4th place. The AIDS virus caused most of the jump, but without this factor, infectious-disease mortality rose 22 percent!

Classes of Infectious Disease	Deaths in 1980	Deaths in 1992
Respiratory Tract Infections	57,000	77,300
Blood Diseases	9,400	33,600
Kidney\Urinary Infections	8,000	19,700
Heart Infections	2,500	12,400
Tuberculosis	2,300	4,000

In the past decades new infections like the AIDS virus have begun killing hundreds of thousands. Older diseases like tuberculosis are now a threat again and bacteria began evolving to defy treatment.

According to Nobel laureate, Joshua Lederberg, *"We have the rumbles of volcanoes that are going to erupt. We don't know if the eruptions will be tomorrow or... in 30 years, but the scene is set for any number of outbreaks. Our technical abilities could give us the necessary defenses."*

STROKE

What is a stroke?

A stroke occurs when the flow of blood going to the brain is blocked by a blood clot or other serious medical problems that impede the vital blood flow to the brain. A blood clot that impedes or stops the needed flow of blood to the brain also blocks the much needed oxygen required for life of the brain. When the brain doesn't get the blood and nourishment it needs, brain cells die. Once these brain cells are gone they're gone forever. Even damaged brain cells can't heal themselves. Atherosclerosis is the leading cause of stroke. See atherosclerosis in Section 26.

What is the stroke mortality rate compared with heart disease and cancer?

Stroke is the fourth leading cause of death behind heart disease, cancer, and infectious diseases. Each year, approximately 500,000 Americans suffer from a stroke. Approximately 33 percent die and the remaining percentage who survive undergo the long process of rehabilitation which is often unsuccessful.

What are some important factors leading to stroke?

Factors that increase the chances of stroke are:

- Alcohol abuse
- Cocaine abuse
- High fat diet
- High cholesterol diet
- Sedentary lifestyle (couch potato type)
- Smoking

If you have one or more of these unhealthy and possibly illegal traits, seek help immediately.

SECTION 07 - High Blood Pressure The Silent Killer!

What is high blood pressure?

High blood pressure is also called hypertension. When your blood pressure remains high no matter what time of day, your activity, or your mood this is good indicator that you may have high blood pressure/hypertension. Approximately 125 million Americans have high blood pressure. Many Americans have NO IDEA their blood pressure is DANGEROUSLY HIGH!

What are the causes of high blood pressure?

High blood pressure may increase with age. It tends to run in the family. It's twice as common in blacks than in whites. It's more common in men than in women. Overweight people are more apt to have hypertension than non-obese people. If one or both of your parents have high blood pressure, you should have your blood pressure checked as soon as possible and several times a year. Many clinics, hospitals, and medical mobile vans offer free checkups. Read Section 25 for healthy sources you SHOULD refer to for additional information. Call your local medical clinics and hospitals for their next scheduled free medical checkups.

What are the symptoms of high blood pressure?

There really are no symptoms of high blood pressure. Meaning you can't feel it, taste it, or notice signs directly indicating that you have high blood pressure.

That is why high blood pressure is called *"THE SILENT KILLER."* If you have high blood pressure you can feel just fine, just great one moment, then POW!!!

I don't have serious high blood pressure now, but how can I prevent it in the future?

Make an appointment with your doctor for starters. Your doctor spent years learning about the medical aspects of the body and only your doctor can legally advise and prescribe drugs (if necessary) for patients with dangerously high blood pressure. Watch your weight. High blood pressure is common in overweight people. Get on a low fat diet to lower your cholesterol so blood flow is less restrictive through your cardiovascular system. Watch your sodium intake and follow your doctor's advice on exercise.

SECTION 08 - Cholesterol, Are You All Sludged-Up?

What is cholesterol and where does it come from?

Cholesterol is a waxy fat-like substance that is made by the liver. However, animal products make-up most of the cholesterol in today's American diet and poor eating habits. Cholesterol's job is to carry digested fat from the liver through your blood vessels to all parts of the body for energy and repair. Fat cannot travel through your blood vessels on its own because fat doesn't mix with water and water is a major ingredient in blood. Cholesterol also carries fat to fat storage sites like the hips, belly, and buttocks. Cholesterol also comes from the foods that you eat. Read the Nutritional Facts on all food items that you anticipate purchasing. Pay strict attention to the SATURATED FAT and CHOLESTEROL content. Purchase food products with the least amount of SATURATED FAT, CHOLESTEROL, SUGAR, and SODIUM. Remember to do the math as instructed in Section 02 and find the TRUE fat content! Re-read Section 01 - EAT THE RIGHT STUFF!!

Cholesterol and its effects on your life?

The National Cholesterol Education Program recommends that everyone over 20 years of age should have their cholesterol level tested and aim for a measurement of 200 mg/dl or less. A high cholesterol reading may lead to heart attacks while a lower cholesterol reading puts you at a much lower risk.

According to the National Center for Health Statistics, 50 percent of Americans ages 20 through 74 have borderline to high cholesterol levels. Only an estimated 30 percent of those know their cholesterol level.

Americans come in second behind people in Finland that have the highest cholesterol average of 265. Cholesterol: You can't see it. You can't feel it. You can't hear it. You can feel fine while your high cholesterol is sneaking up on you. High cholesterol leads to heart attacks, heart disease, stroke, and other cardiovascular diseases!

Are there different types of cholesterol?

The liver puts cholesterol into packages called lipoproteins. Lipoproteins are made from lipids (fat and cholesterol) and protein. There are three kinds of lipoprotein packages. These three lipoprotein packages are called Very Low-Density Lipoprotein (VLDL), Low-Density Lipoprotein (LDL) and High-Density Lipoprotein (HDL). The VLDL, LDL, and HDL each have their own special job.

VLDL -- Once you eat fat, it is digested and absorbed in the small intestine and is then sent to the liver for processing into VLDL packaging and transportation throughout the body. VLDL carries the fat from the liver to all parts of your body. Again, fat cannot travel through your blood vessels on its own because fat doesn't mix with water and water is a major ingredient in blood.

LDL -- Once VLDL drops off the fat throughout your body, it becomes empty VLDL or better yet LDL. LDL becomes *"BAD CHOLESTEROL"* because pieces of LDL become stuck along blood vessel walls on its way back to the liver to be reprocessed to new VLDL or broken down and excreted as waste. These pieces of LDL become stuck narrowing the blood vessel walls. This leads to high blood pressure. You already read the section on High Blood Pressure - The Silent Killer - so you know the consequences of high blood pressure.

HDL -- HDL is called the *"GOOD CHOLESTEROL."* HDL's job is to find LDL that is stuck to your blood vessels, liberate the LDL from the blood vessel, and take it back to the liver to be reprocessed to new VLDL or broken down and excreted as waste. You might think of HDLs as being the *"arterial vacuum cleaner"* in the blood! HDL levels below 35 increase the risk of heart disease, while levels above 65 strongly reduce the risk of heart disease. You can increase the GOOD CHOLESTEROL, HDL, by simply exercising (frequent, regular exercise)! According to Larry Gibbons, M.D., of the Cooper Clinic in Dallas, Texas, *"HDL is the single most important predictor of heart disease among the lipid fractions."*

How can I lower my cholesterol?

According to the American Heart Association you should get only 30% of all your calories from fat. However, Dr. Sheldon Saul Hendler, author of The Doctor's Vitamin and Mineral Encyclopedia states that ideal cholesterol lowering diet *"consists of 20% calories from fat."* Dr. Dean Ornish, of the University of California at San Diego states that a cholesterol lowering diet should consist of 10 percent calories from fat.

Dr. Ornish's Heart Disease Reversal studies have demonstrated that at this low intake level of fat one can literally unplug arteries and UNDO heart disease. The 8-Week Cholesterol Cure by Robert E. Kowalski, is highly recommended reading for anyone that desires to lower their cholesterol level and lose weight. Here's one testimony from this amazing book: *"My blood cholesterol dropped from 288 to 150 in seven weeks. When I told my cardiologist this, his response was unbelievable!"* Diet is instrumental in lowering your cholesterol. So EAT THE RIGHT STUFF and read *"The 8-Week Cholesterol Cure."* (see References)

SECTION 09 - Free Radicals And Antioxidants!

What are these things called Free Radicals and what do they do?
Historical research on free radicals goes way back, but I'll only go back as far as 1954. In 1954, the destructive power of free radicals on the human body was recognized. The blame was the main support of life on Earth - OXYGEN! Breathing pure oxygen for as little as six hours causes chest soreness, sore throats, and coughing. During the 1940's, the medical establishment was puzzled over a form of blindness called retrolental fibroplasia which appeared in premature infants. Two American scientists (Rebecca Gershman & Daniel L. Gilbert) and others determined that the source of the problem was the incubators where the premature babies were placed which had a higher oxygen content than the air you and I breath. The premature babies were exposed to oxygen free radicals. During the following years, four destructive forms of oxygen were identified. Two are true free radicals (unpaired electron in molecular orbit) called hydroxyl radical and superoxide radical. The other two other forms of destructive oxygen are called oxygen singlet and hydrogen peroxide, *"non-radical reactive oxygen species."* These four free radicals can do significant damage to the human body. Free radicals are linked to fifty medical problems including various forms of cancer, premature aging, heart disease, cataracts, and even AIDS!

How are renegade free radicals linked to Coronary Artery Disease?
Coronary artery disease is the major cause of heart attacks. Heart attacks occur when atherosclerosis is present in the vital coronary arteries. Remember that once VLDL drops-off the fat throughout your body it becomes empty VLDL or better yet LDL. LDL becomes *"BAD CHOLESTEROL"* because pieces of LDL become stuck along blood vessel walls on its way back to the liver to be reprocessed to new VLDL or broken down and excreted as waste. These pieces of LDL become stuck narrowing the blood vessel walls. LDL (low density lipoproteins\bad cholesterol) has been marked as the main fault of cholesterol-clogging atherosclerosis. Once pieces of LDL become stuck inside the walls of the blood vessels, these LDL pieces oxidize because of their exposure to free radicals. White blood cells called macrophages attempt to remove these pieces of oxidized LDL by eating them up. After eating the pieces of LDL, the macrophages swell up because they are unable to get rid of the cholesterol. This leads to thickening of the artery wall and narrowing of the coronary arteries.

How are renegade free radicals linked to Cancer?

Free radicals are triggered by factors such as cigarette smoke, air pollution, ultraviolet radiation and possibly stress and overtraining. Free radicals penetrate deep inside cells and damage the nucleus which carries the DNA. DNA is the genetic code of the cell. This cell may grow out of control with possible malignant lesions and tumors. Renegade free radicals have been implicated to cancers of the cervix, colon, esophagus, lungs, prostate, skin, and stomach.

Antioxidants are well documented to offset the health threats of damaging free radicals.

What are antioxidants?

An antioxidant is any agent that prevents a substance from reacting with oxygen, helping to counteract the reactions caused by peroxides or oxygen in the body. An antioxidant is defined chemically as a natural or synthetic substance used to help prevent or delay deterioration through the action of oxygen. Antioxidants protect against cancer and aging.

What are the benefits of antioxidants?

According to Dr. Kenneth H. Cooper author of Antioxidant Revolution the benefits of antioxidants are:

- Increased protection from many forms of cancer.
- Stronger defense against cardiovascular disease, such as atherosclerosis, heart attacks, and strokes.
- The preservation of your eyesight through the prevention of cataracts.
- A delay in the onset of premature aging.
- A more powerful immune system.
- A decreased risk of early Parkinson's disease and a host of other major advantages for your health.

Where can I obtain authentic antioxidant supplements?

I dedicated an entire section to one of a very few sources of authentic antioxidant products.

Go to Section 12 and read *Pycnogenol The Antioxidant Of Choice.*

SECTION 10 – ALCOHOLISM, THE SOBERING FACTS

What is Alcohol?

Alcohol is a drug. Like sedatives, alcohol depresses the central nervous system and is the major psychoactive ingredient in wine, beer, and distilled liquors.

What effect does alcohol have on my mind, body and health?

In small quantities, alcohol has a tranquilizing effect on most people, although it appears to stimulate others. Alcohol first acts on those parts of the brain which affect self-control and other learned behaviors. Lowered self-control may lead to the aggressive behavior associated with some people who drink.

Individual, physical, mental, and environmental factors may determine how people react to alcohol or any other psychoactive drug.

Can alcohol kill?

It sure can. A large quantity of alcohol like a pint of whiskey or less, consumed at once can interfere with the part of the brain that controls breathing. This respiratory failure can lead to death.

Delirium tremens which is the most extreme manifestation of alcohol withdrawal, can lead to death.

On the average, heavy drinkers shorten their life span by about 10 years!

I just drink a few times a year on special occasions and such. Can I become dependent on alcohol?

Yes, if drinkers see alcohol as an escape from the problems and stresses of everyday life. They may begin to depend on the drug (alcohol in this case) for relief. Repeated drinking produces tolerance to the drug's effects and dependence. The body then needs alcohol to function. Once a drinker is dependent upon alcohol, they experience withdrawal symptoms when they stop drinking. In some serious cases, hospitalization may be necessary to ensure a safe withdrawal. If you must drink, be a sensible moderate drinker.

OK, I may suffer from alcoholism, I might be a an alcoholic. What is alcoholism and am I an alcoholic?

Alcoholism is a treatable illness, which is characterized by the drinker's consistent inability to choose to stop drinking when they have obviously had enough. It is more than enough when a person becomes drunk. It is more than enough when drinking has a negative impact on families, friends and your job. By this criteria, more than 10 million Americans are problem drinkers or alcoholics.

The length of time a person has been drinking and how much that person drinks is not as important in determining alcoholism as what happens when a person drinks. An alcoholic's drinking reflects repeated problems that affect family, job, and self. If left untreated, alcoholism progresses resulting in death or insanity.

I may be an alcoholic. What can I do?

The most difficult step is for the alcoholic to admit the need for help. Most alcoholics require professional counseling or care in either an inpatient or an outpatient treatment program. Involvement with Alcoholics Anonymous is also highly advisable.

What are some symptoms for alcoholism?

Do you or does someone you know...

- Drink to relieve shyness, fear or inadequacy?
- Find personal relationships more difficult to maintain?
- Find your drinking is harmful or worrying your family?
- Find your efficiency and ambition decreasing due to drinking?
- Find yourself more moody, jealous, or irritable after drinking?
- Have loss of memory while or after drinking?
- Like to drink alone frequently?
- Lose time from work due to drinking?
- Need a drink at a definite time daily?
- Need a drink the *"morning after?"*

If you answered *"YES"* to one or more of these questions, a professional evaluation by a substance abuse counselor is recommended.

Alcohol abuse is nothing but BAD NEWS! Are there any positive effects of moderate and responsible alcohol consumption?

The French have high-risk diets that are rich in saturated fats, yet their heart disease is 2.5 times LOWER than the United States! WHY? Call it the French Factor or whatever you want. The French love their red wine! One healthy ingredient in the French diet is a substance called Flavonoids. Flavonoids are natural compounds found in red wine and in almost all fruits and vegetables. Flavonoids have been noted to help protect against heart disease and possibly cancer!

WARNING: The French may have a lower rate of heart disease because of their consumption of red wine (flavonoids), but on the other hand they have a high rate of cirrhosis of the liver. DO NOT abuse alcohol!

SECTION 11 - TOXINS, CHEMICALS, FOOD ADDITIVES, CREATURES, & GASES ARE INVADING YOUR HOME AND YOUR HEALTH RIGHT NOW!

Did you know that you spend most of your life in your home? You are living in your nice comfortable home and you never give a second thought that your own home IS endangering your health right now. Millions of Americans are needlessly suffering from many maladies because they're not aware of the many threats to their health in their own home. Once you're aware of these health threats, there are ways to neutralize, control and\or avoid these threats in the future. This section will cover the unknown health hazards within your own home. Twenty-four hours a day, YOU ARE EXPOSED to one, a few, or all of the health hazards listed below and are probably not aware of it. I will expose each health hazard as well as give you a solution(s). You may be surprised how your health may improve once these health hazards are removed or controlled in your home environment. You may also be investing in your HEALTHY FUTURE by knowing about these home health hazards and taking proper action.

The health hazards that we'll cover in this section are:

- ALUMINUM
- ASBESTOS
- CARBON MONOXIDE
- DERMATOPHAGOIDES
- ELECTROMAGNETIC FIELDS (EMF)
- ENVIRONMENTAL TOBACCO
- FIVE DEADLY WHITES
- SMOKE (ETS)
- HOUSEDUST & MORE
- HOUSEHOLD CONSUMABLES & HOME CONSTRUCTION MATERIALS
- LEAD
- MERCURY
- MSG
- RADON GAS
- WATER (polluted)

ALUMINUM

Is aluminum a real threat to my health?

Aluminum has been found to be toxic. Aluminum enters the air, soil, and water. Therefore, small amounts are present in the food we eat. The average person consumes 03 to 10 milligrams of aluminum per day. Recent research has revealed that aluminum is absorbed and accumulated in the body. Many symptoms of aluminum toxicity are similar to those of Alzheimer's disease and osteoporosis.

Aluminum toxicity can lead to:
- aching and weak muscles
- anemia
- colic
- decreased kidney function
- decreased liver function
- extreme nervousness and more…

ASBESTOS

What is asbestos?

Asbestos is any of the fibrous variety of four distinct incombustible, chemical-resistant, silicate minerals, used for fireproofing, electrical insulation, building materials, brake linings, and chemical filters. Asbestos is used in thousands (3,000 to 5,000) of products.

Is asbestos hazardous to my health?

Asbestos is dangerous only when it has deteriorated and its fibers become airborne. These microscopic fibers can't be seen. Once they're inhaled into your lungs, they may cause scarring and cancer. In 1988, EPA risk analysts stated that the United States could expect 131,200 asbestos-related deaths between 1985 and the year 2009.

CARBON MONOXIDE

What is Carbon Monoxide?

Carbon Monoxide is a colorless, odorless, toxic gas that can be emitted by fuel burning appliances if they are not working properly. If fuels do not burn completely or if fuel-burning appliances are not adequately ventilated, harmful amounts of carbon monoxide may accumulate in your home, or automobile.

What happens if I inhale carbon monoxide?

When inhaled, carbon monoxide is absorbed into the bloodstream where it blocks out oxygen to vital tissues and organs. It causes fatigue, headaches, nausea, and vomiting. Prolonged exposure can result in unconsciousness, brain damage, or even death!

According to the Centers for Disease Control and Prevention (CDC) in Atlanta, Georgia, carbon monoxide accounts for approximately one-half of all accidental poisoning deaths in the United States, killing approximately 1,800 Americans each year.

DERMATOPHAGOIDES

What the heck are Dermatophagoides?

Another name for dermatophagoides (skin eater) are house dust mites. The house dust mite wasn't discovered until 1968. House dust mites are microscopic animals. You can't possibly see them. House dust mites belong to the same family as spiders and ticks and have a life span of 02 to 04 months.

How small are house dust mites?

They are so small that as many as 18,000 of these critters can be on one floating speck of dust or as many as 2,000,000 in a double bed!

So what's the problem with the house dust mite?

As I said, a large size adult man or woman sheds about 600,000 skin particles per hour. This flaked human skin is found everywhere in your home and in the work place - places like the carpet, recliner, sofa, bed, and upholstered furniture. That means dust mites are everywhere! Dust mites are eating your shedded skin. They're constantly eating, reproducing, and defecating! A dust mite produces approximately 40 pellets of waste every 24 hours. The waste of the dust mite is the real problem.

ELECTROMAGNETIC FIELDS

What are Electromagnetic Fields (EMF)?

All electric current produces two types of fields: an electric field and a magnetic field. We don't have to worry too much about electric fields because they can easily be blocked by metal or other shielding. A magnetic field is a different story. A magnetic field is able to penetrate most materials therefore able to reach you and possibly do some harm. From here on out, since current produces both electric and magnetic fields, we'll stick to using EMF throughout this topic.

Can EMFs hurt me?

This question Requires Further Intensive Research (RFIR). At this time there is not a conclusive YES or NO answer. Is there a link between EMF's and cancer? The best answer is, it is better to be safe than sorry! Everywhere you go, you may be bombarded by EMF's. Every day you come in contact with appliances that produce EMF's.

ENVIRONMENTAL TOBACCO SMOKE (ETS)

What is Environmental Tobacco Smoke (ETS)?

The Environmental Protection Agency (EPA), in their January 1993 press conference, released their findings and declared ETS a *"Grade A"* human carcinogen-A, designation given to only 10 other potent hazardous compounds, including asbestos, arsenic, benzene, and radon. In other words ETS is a serious threat to your health. If you smoke QUIT!

What can (ETS) do to me and others?

A report issued by the EPA (January 1993) estimates that ETS is responsible for approximately 3,000 lung cancer deaths and another 300,000 lower respiratory-tract infections among children each year. In 1964, the Surgeon General's report declared cigarette smoking a health hazard. In 1986, the Surgeon General's report implicated ETS to lung cancer. Here is some more data:

* 425,000 Americans die every year as a result of diseases related to smoking-140,000 die from lung cancer.

FIVE DEADLY WHITES

What are the Five Deadly Whites (FDWs)?

The five deadly whites are (listed in order as the most dangerous threat to your health): Meat, Dairy, Salt, Sugar, and White Flour.

- **Meat** - Meat contains fat and fat is already linked to many cancers, heart disease, stroke, and diabetes. Meat eaters consume over 50 pounds of fat (cholesterol) each year!

- **Dairy** - Pasteurized milk changes the calcium to an inorganic form which can not be assimilated by your body. Animal products are noted to be sources of LDL (bad cholesterol).

- **Salt** - Your body needs sodium but the sodium chloride (table salt) may be toxic to your body! For more information and a far superior sodium product see Whole Salt in Section 14!

- **Sugar** - Sugar is linked to a wide variety of health problems and noted to hinder your immune system. In Section 26, I annotated an alternative called stevia.

- **White Flour** -- White flour is missing most of the good ingredients prior to its processing. It's bleached, synthetic   Vitamins added, and it's called *"enriched."* Remember the saying   I gave you in Section 01 concerning bread *"The whiter the bread, the sooner you're dead!"*

***HOUSE DUST & MORE ***

What is house dust?

There is much more to house dust than dirt. House dust is composed of many particles. According to Alfred V. Zamm, M.D., F.A.C.A., F.A.C.P., author of Why Your House May Endanger Your Health, house dust is comprised of three categories: Plant, Animal, and Manmade. Below is a list of those particles found in each category.

PLANT	ANIMAL	MANMADE
Cellulose:	Fragments:	Acrilan
cotton	ants	Cigarette Smoke
kapok	beetles	Dacron
linen	cockroaches	Fiberglass
wood	feathers	Fireplace soot
	fleas	Lycra
Mold Spores	mosquitoes	Nylon
	moths	Orlon
Cellulose:	Fragments:	Acrilan
Pollen	silverfish	Paint
	spiders	Plastic
	Furs	Rayon
	Hair	Rubber
	Horsehair	Spandex
	House Dustmites	
	Mohair	
	Pet Dander	
	Rabbit Fur	
	Silk	

Some physicians are now viewing house dust as an *"occupational hazard"* for the homemaker. When attempting to clean the home, the homemaker stirs-up enormous quantities of house dust and the homemaker, as well as family members, are inhaling millions of these pollutants! According to one study, an average six-room home in a city or in the suburbs accumulates forty pounds of dust a year! The plant particles come from everything from clothes, sofa, carpet, and hats.

HOUSEHOLD CONSUMABLES & HOME CONSTRUCTION MATERIALS

The household is overwhelmed by unhealthy man-made chemicals that you use when cleaning your house, doing laundry, and other household chores. Even your house itself may be constructed of unhealthy materials. Vapors in the house from evaporating chemicals and heating and cooking appliances are also possible health hazards to your home.

I'll try to expose some of these health hazards and give solutions.

Can household consumables and home construction materials really pose a threat to my health?

Based on surveys begun in 1979, the Environmental Protection Agency's (EPA), Total Exposure Assessment Methodology (TEAM) study was designed to document and characterize actual human exposures to the family of substances known as Volatile Organic Compounds (VOC) which are found in household consumables (aerosols, cleaning compounds, and adhesives) and home construction materials.

What are Volatile Organic Chemicals (VOC)?

VOC's are a class of carbon-based chemicals that volatilize or evaporate at room temperature. Sources of VOCs are solvents, organochlorines, and phenols. VOCs, through research have indicated that they cause acute and chronic health effects which may include blurred vision, dizziness, euphoria, fatigue, headaches, irritations of the eyes, nose & throat, joint pain, numbness in extremities and weakness. The most common VOC found in indoor air is formaldehyde. Sources of some VOC's are:

- **Solvents:** Adhesives, cleaners, cosmetics (containing: benzene, toluene, methyl, & ethyl compounds), degreasers, laquers, paints, and strippers.

- **Organochlorines:** Cleaning agents, pesticides, and preservatives such as carbon tetrachloride, chlorobenzene, chlordane, heptachlor, hexachlorophene, pentachlorophenol, 1,1,1- trichloroethane, and trichloroethane. PCB's and vinyl chloride are also included.

- Phenols: Air fresheners, antiseptics, cleaners, coal tar, disinfectants, glues, mouthwashes, perfumes, petroleum compounds, plastics, polishes, and waxes.

LEAD POISONING

What is lead poisoning?

Lead is undoubtedly one of the most toxic metal contaminants! It is a poison that is retained in the bones, brain, central nervous system, glands, and hair. Sources of lead are: antique pewter, bone meal, canned fruit (lead soldered cans leaches out and absorbed by the fruit), ceramic glazes, crystal wine glasses, decanters, some domestic and imported wines, garden vegetables (depending on the soil), imported ceramic pottery, glass artwork, insecticides, lead-acid batteries used in autos, lead-based paint, lead dust, leaded gasoline, lead pipes, metallic fishing weights, piping with solder, tobacco, water (supplied through lead piping), and wine bottle foils. The EPA banned the use of lead in nearly all paints made in the United States, but by that time the United States Public Health Service estimated that varying levels of lead paint was applied to walls, woodwork and windows of approximately 57 million American homes and 75 percent of all houses built before 1980.

What can lead poisoning do to my health?

Lead accumulates in the body. The primary health risk of lead is damage to the brain and nervous system. Other toxic amounts of lead can damage the heart, kidneys, and liver. Lead poisoning causes days of severe gastrointestinal colic, gums turning blue, and a person may experience muscle weakness. Chronic lead poisoning causes anemia, impotence in men, high blood pressure, infertility, and reproductive disorders. High levels of lead in the body have been linked to hyperactivity. Lead poisoning can eventually lead to blindness, insanity, loss of memory, mental disturbances, mental retardation, and paralysis of the extremities. Even minute amounts of lead have been noted to cause learning disabilities, lowered Intelligence Quotient (IQ), speech impairments, and other neuropsychological problems.

MERCURY

What is mercury?

Mercury was discovered approximately 5,000 years ago. Because of its silvery appearance, it was nicknamed *"quick silver."* Mercury is a heavy metal, meaning it has a high molecular weight and characterized by its ability to produce toxic reactions in living organisms. Mercury is a heavy silver-white poisonous metallic element that is liquid at room temperature. Mercury has not been found to be beneficial to your health.

Mercury is used in drugs, medicines, widely used in industry, and may be used at your dental office in the form of amalgam fillings!

Am I exposed to mercury?

Mercury is found in the air, food, and water. You may even be exposed to mercury at the dental office. Mercury is used in dentistry, drugs, and industry. The following is a partial list where mercury is used and found (contamination):

- Agriculture
- Air (contamination)
- Amalgam filling (dentistry)
- Batteries
- Beverages (contamination)
- Cosmetics - skin creams, hair dyes....
- Detonator in explosive caps (salt form)
- Drugs (salt form)
- Fungicides (salt form)
- Insecticides (salt form)
- Lamps
- Light switches
- Paint pigments (salt form)
- Processed food (contamination)
- Seafood (contamination)
- Street lights
- Thermometers
- Water - oceans, lakes, rivers... (contamination)

RADON GAS

What is Radon Gas and how does it get in my home?

Radon is a colorless, tasteless, and odorless gas that seeps into some homes as uranium deteriorates in the soil below the foundation. Radon is the decaying product of radium and uranium, present in nearly all rocks and soils on Mother Earth including granite, shale, and phosphate. Concentrations of radon in indoor air are expressed as picouries per liter (pCi/L) of air, a measure of the rate of decaying uranium.

The EPA believes no level of radon is safe. Guidelines recommend homes with levels of 4.0 pCi/L or higher should be modified to reduce radon concentrations. This deteriorating uranium could be almost anywhere. Sources of radon may be found in well water and building materials. However, a principal source of radon is soil gases seeping into a home from cracks, holes in the foundation walls, floors, pipes, sumps, and other openings. By design, tightly-insulated and poorly ventilated homes can draw radon gas into the home because of the *"negative"* air pressure.

Can Radon Gas hurt me?

In 1984, a worker at the Limerick Nuclear Power Plant in Pennsylvania inexplicably set off the radiation-checkpoint alarms within the plant. Reactor technicians couldn't make sense of it because this employee's job as a plant engineer required no contact with radioactive materials. When officials checked this employee's home, they found the culprit.

It was radiation from radon gas seeping into his home and being carried into the plant on the employee's clothes. The employee's house was built on top of a uranium-rich geologic formation known as the Reading Prong that goes through Northeastern United States. The employee and his family were being bathed in radon levels nearly ONE THOUSAND times higher than those radon levels deemed safe under federal guidelines. The employee and his family were exposed to high radon levels equivalent to smoking HUNDREDS OF CIGARETTES A DAY and receiving more than HALF A MILLION CHEST X-RAYS A YEAR. This case drew national headlines which prompted federal regulators to begin assessing the wider public health risk of the naturally occurring gas called radon.

This high level of radon may not be common to households across the United States, but even a small level of radon may be hazardous to your health! Location of your home or rented apartment may make a difference in your health. Before you purchase that house or move into that rental apartment, ask about recent radon testing.

According to researchers, long-term exposure to high levels of radon gas may cause lung cancer. Radon kills approximately 14,000 Americans per year. According to EPA projections, almost one out of every fifteen homes exceed the 4.0 pCi/L guideline. Radon may be the second leading cause of lung cancer.

WATER*

There's plenty of water. Is there a concern for clean, drinkable water?
Water is approximately 03 billion years old. Mother Nature recycles water through evaporation by the power of the sun, condensation (which is the formation of clouds) and finally through precipitation via rain, snow, sleet or hail. Your body discharges approximately 03 quarts of water per day, therefore, you must drink at least 03 quarts of water per day to at least compensate for water discharge. Even when you exhale, you're discharging water. Most people get their water from the faucet in the home or work-place.

Due to industrialization, the use of a multitude of chemicals and pesticides, many water resources are polluted and will remain polluted in your lifetime no matter what Mother Nature does to recycle the water. Clean water resources aren't as plentiful as they were years ago. Approximately 900 Americans die from drinking contaminated water and hundreds of thousands of Americans become ill each year. According to the Environmental Protection Agency (EPA), many outdated water treatment systems throughout the United States can't eliminate chemicals and deadly bacteria in the water being treated.

According to the EPA, 1,000 water treatment systems that service 13,000,000 people are outdated. According to the EPA, in 1994, approximately 30,000,000 Americans (12% of the population) were served drinking water that violated 01 or more public health hazards! More than 100 waterborne disease outbreaks have been reported since 1986 which caused many deaths and many more to become sick. In 1993, cryptosporidium parvum, a waterborne parasite, caused 104 deaths and caused more than 400,000 people to become sick in Milwaukee!

In the United States, approximately 900 people die each year drinking contaminated water and another million people become ill. The Federal Government - Environmental Protection Agency (EPA) warned that the nations' water treatments are in bad shape. 09 out of 10 water treatment facilities are out-of-date!

****Working Has A Toxic Effect****

Am I exposed to any toxins at my job?
The following is a list of common jobs and possible toxins that workers may be exposed to at any time.

Aircraft Workers -- Chemicals in chlorinated solvents, hydraulic fluids, lubricating oils, paints & paint thinners, plastics and resins, radiation, and welding fumes.

Airline Pilots and Crew -- Formaldehyde in upholstery fabric, fuel, oils, and Environmental Tobacco Smoke (ETS) - depending on their location and restrictions on the use of tobacco products.

Auto Mechanics -- Asbestos dust from brakes & auto parts, benzene from carburetor cleaner, brake fluids, carbon monoxide, gasoline, graphite, grease, kerosene, lubricating oils, and soldering metals.

Bakers -- Additives in foods, disinfectants, flour dust, fluorocarbons from refrigeration, fumigants, fungicides, and gas from ovens.

Barbers and Beauticians -- Chemicals in cosmetics, disinfectants, dyes, hair preparations, nail products, perfumes, and sprays.

Brewers -- Carbon dioxide and carbon monoxide, hydrogen fluoride and hydrogen sulfide and sulfur dioxide are all given off during the fermentation process.

Butchers and Meat Workers -- Antibiotics, detergents, fungicides, herbicides, pesticides from grasses fed to animals, hormones to fatten animals, and vinyl fumes from meat wrapping.

Carpenters and Construction Workers -- Adhesives, arsenic in paint, glass, wallpaper, asbestos, insulation, lead, oils, solvents, stains, and varnishes.

Ceramic Workers -- Natural gas, acetylene, arsenic, asbestos, beryllium, cadmium, chromium, cobalt, fluoride, lead, mercury, nickel, selenium, uranium compounds, and zinc.

SECTION 12 – Pycnogenol The Antioxidant Of Choice

Every second of every day our body cells are exposed to alcohol, exhaust fumes, pesticides, pollution, processed foods, preservatives, poor nutrition, stress, tobacco smoke, toxins, and x-rays.

These environmental hazards and your own lifestyle choices cause arthritis, bruising, cancer, clogged arteries, heart disease, lack of energy, liver damage, mental deterioration, poor circulation, premature aging, and susceptibility to sports injuries.

One way our body protects itself against pollutants is by forming antioxidants in the form of super oxide dismutase (SOD). The most common antioxidants found in foods are Vitamins A, C, E, and selenium. However, the continual bombardment of stress, environmental pollution, and food processing destroy antioxidants allowing the body to be more susceptible to disease and ill health. Your body already has a difficult time producing enough antioxidants to combat the multitude of contaminants it's exposed to every second!

Antioxidants can help ALZHEIMER'S DISEASE, ARTHRITIS, CANCER, HEART DISEASE, JET LAG, PROSTATE, and STROKE.

There are 60 chronic degenerative diseases that science knows of that are caused by free radicals.

Professor Jacques Masquelier of the University of Bordeaux, France was granted a U.S. patent for Pycnogenol (a registered trademark of Horphag Overseas Limited). Pycnogenol is a natural plant product made from the bark of the European coastal pine, Pinus Maritima. Pycnogenol is the most POWERFUL antioxidant today and acts as a protector against environmental toxins! Research has demonstrated that Pycnogenol is 50 times more effective than Vitamin E and 20 times more powerful than Vitamin C! Studies show that Pycnogenol is rapidly absorbed and distributed throughout the body within 20 minutes. Pycnogenol helps activate Vitamin C and has it working before it leaves your body. Pycnogenol is being used in France, Finland, Holland, Germany, Switzerland, and now the United States.

Pycnogenol is a perfect weapon to prevent ill health and premature aging. Using supplements to increase the intake of antioxidants can build the body's defenses and may slow down the aging process. Pycnogenol is an effective antioxidant that is possibly one of the MOST POWERFUL FREE RADICAL SCAVENGERS AVAILABLE!

The following are only 40% of some of the documented health benefits from the research of Dr. Richard Passwater, Dr. Jacques Masquelier, Dr. Morton Walker, Pasteur & Huntington Institutes, and seven other leading Universities in Europe.

- Decreases Allergies\Hay fever
- Enhance Immune Resistance
- Helps Alzheimer's
- Helps Asthma\Bronchitis
- Helps Diabetes
- Improves Circulation
- Improves Joint Flexibility
- Improves Skin Smoothness
- Increases Energy, Less Fatigue
- Lowers Cholesterol
- Prevents Ulcer Formation
- Prevents Fat Formation\Cellulitis
- Prevents Wrinkling of the Skin
- Reduces Arthritis Pain
- Reduces Blood Pressure
- Reduces Infection\Flu\Cold
- Reduces Menopause\PMS\Cramps
- Reduces Risk of Cancer
- Reduces Risk of Phlebitis
- Reduces Risk of Stroke
- Reduces Stress\Depression
- Reduces Varicose Veins
- Repairs Atherosclerosis

- Resists Mutagen Attacks
- Resists Oxidized LDL
- Retards Aging
- Strengthens Capillaries

What is Pycnogenol and what can it do for me?

Pycnogenol is an extract from the maritime pine consisting of proanthocyanidins and water-soluble nutrients. Pycnogenol, a specific blend of bioflavonoids (patented), a *"super protector nutrient"* is a made up of powerful antioxidant nutrients for use to scavenge free radicals. The mixture of nutrients can help you live better longer, stay healthier, and appear more youthful. Pycnogenol is noted to protect you from approximately 80 diseases, including arthritis, cancer, heart disease, and most non-germ diseases which are linked to the deleterious chemical action of free radicals.

SECTION 13 - The Amazing Qualities Of Garlic And Vinegar!

Garlic and vinegar are being recognized as having disease-preventing and miraculous health-building powers. These two wonders are being used by more and more people throughout the world every day. Garlic and vinegar have been recognized by the scientific world as having disease-fighting and powerful germ-killing qualities. Garlic and vinegar are able to spur the immune system to resist and overcome common and uncommon conditions.

Do you need an antidote to a virus? Do you want to reduce blood pressure? Do you want to wash-out oxidated LDL (Low Density Lipo-protein) and other debris? Do you want to stimulate your cardiovascular system? Do you want to overcome bacterial infection? Scientists have found garlic and vinegar helpful in cleansing the blood, as well as debilitating disorders as colitis, gastritis, respiratory problems, and even cancer.

GARLIC

What can you tell me about garlic; what makes it work, and why does it work?
As early as 1500 B.C., it is noted that Egyptians listed 22 garlic prescriptions for a variety of ailments including heart problems, headaches, and physical weakness. Hippocrates, a Greek physician, recommended garlic as a remedy. Chinese Herbal Code indicates that aged garlic has been used for heart problems for over 1,000 years. Garlic was used by folk healers to fight infection, cleanse the system of harmful substances, reduce high blood pressure, and stimulate the immune system. Recently, the medical field has rediscovered the value and benefits of natural medicines from the plant world. One herb from the plant field noted for its wide range of therapeutic qualities is GARLIC. Garlic research has focused on many areas including:
- Anti-bacterial effects
- Anti-viral effects
- Antioxidant
- Blood pressure
- Cancer prevention and care
- Cardio vascular care.

- Cholesterol
- Memory improvement

VINEGAR

In 5,000 B.C., Babylonians fermented the fruits of the date palm. This date vinegar was credited for having superior healing qualities. Vinegar is even mentioned in the Bible (four times in the Old Testament and four times in the New Testament). Claims of curative and restorative powers of apple cider vinegar are legendary. This fabulous liquid is associated with believers who say it can lengthen life, improve hearing, mental powers, and vision. Vinegar has been used thousands of years for folk medicine, hair, and skin care.

Vinegar comes from the French word *"vinaigre"* -- Vin for wine and Aigre for sour, thus wine that has gone sour. Vinegar is an acid liquid made from beer, cider, and wine by a means called acetous fermentation meaning alcohol mixes with oxygen in the air. The alcohol is changed into acetic acid and water. The acetic acid gives vinegar it's unique tart taste. Vinegar contents has the basic nutrients of the original food from which it was made. Here's an example: Apple Cider Vinegar (ACV) has beta carotene, pectin, and potassium. All which are very beneficial for your health as annotated in this book.

What does Apple Cider Vinegar (ACV) have in it, that makes it so beneficial for our mind and body?

ACV is packed with amino acids, healthful enzymes and trace elements. It contains more than thirty needed nutrients, a dozen minerals, and several Vitamins, essential acids, and enzymes. ACV has a tart taste and a germ killing acid and pectin for those heart healthy concerned.

ACV is a great source of calcium, chlorine, fluorine, iron, magnesium, phosphorus, potassium, silicon, sodium, and sulfur. The body requires 22 essential minerals for health and 19 of them are found in ACV! Potassium in ACV is known for its aid to overall circulation.

SECTION 14 - Vitamins, Minerals, Amazing Supplements, And Other Health Benefitting Information You Should Know About For Your Healthy Future!

This section covers Vitamins, Minerals, and other unknown supplements that are addressed throughout this book, but is not a complete list. Mega-doses of Minerals, Vitamins, and other healthy supplements can't compensate for poor eating habits and will not compensate your diet for the lack of fiber and those newly discovered phytochemicals! So EAT THE RIGHT STUFF, take your Vitamins, minerals, and supplements and stay away from EXCESS salt\sodium, saturated fat, sugar, all tobacco products, alcohol, and exercise regularly (see your physician)! Browse throughout Section 25, for a wide variety of health enhancing companies with healthy products.

AMINO ACIDS: Amino acids are the *"building blocks"* of protein. The 22 known amino acids are vital to your health because they help build, repair, renew, and provide a source of energy. If any amino acid is low or missing, the effectiveness of all the others will be reduced and must be obtained from food or supplements. Of the 22 known amino acids, eight of them are not manufactured by the body. Here are seven of them: Isoleucine, Leucine, Lysine, Phenylalanine, Theronine, Tryptophan, and Valine. Here are a few amino acids and what they do for you:

Carnitine: Carnitine can help in the breakdown of fats so that they can be used as energy for the body. Carnitine is a factor in making muscles operate at their best possible strength level.

Taurine: Taurine could possibly help retard the development of hypertension. Taurine helps strengthen brain-wave patterns. Taurine helps increase the white blood cells that fight infections. Follow the recommended dosage and instructions from the label and as per your doctor's instructions.

BEE POLLEN: Did you know honey bee pollen is one of the world's oldest health foods for the athlete? Bee Pollen is a very fine powder making up the male element of flower. Those busy bees gather pollen in microscopic amounts and carry it to their hive. Bees instinctively collect the most nutritious and healthy bee pollen.

BIOTIN: A B Vitamin that may work synergistically* and alone to lower blood sugar. A 1985 study revealed that diabetic participants who were given a daily dose of biotin (16mg) demonstrated lower blood sugar levels while the other half, - the placebo group, their blood sugar rose! This micronutrient may help ameliorate a diabetic condition!

BROMELAIN: Bromelain is a natural enzyme found in pineapples. This nutrient increases the body's ability to break down fats and protein promoting body metabolism!
Follow the recommended dosage and instructions from the label and as per your doctor's instructions.

CALCIUM: Calcium is vital to your health. Ninety-nine (99) percent of all calcium is found in our bones. A lack of this very important nutrient can lead to loss of height, teeth, back pain, and weak porous bones that can crack or break. As your body matures, the demand for calcium increases.

Calcium keeps the teeth strong, helps the body utilize iron, and aids the passage of nutrients. Lack of exercise, stress, aspirin, antibiotics, excess intake of fats, and mineral oil can have leave you lacking this very important mineral.
Follow the recommended dosage and instructions from the label and as per your doctor's instructions.

CATALYST WATER -- WATER THAT HEALS!: Water is the most important biological factor sustaining living organisms. Water molecules improve and speed up cell movement, and aid nutrients moving into and out of living organisms cells.

Catalyst water is pure ordinary water which has been treated with a catalyst. The catalyst appears to change the molecular structure of the water, making the molecules smaller.

When this happens, the water becomes more penetrable, and anything dissolved in the water like beneficial nutrients from food, minerals, and Vitamins is more readily absorbed into our bodies.

CHROMIUM PICOLINATE: Chromium picolinate is an essential trace mineral which facilitates the action of insulin, glucose, and protein and fat metabolism. Chromium picolinate is noted to enhance the body's sensitivity to insulin and may reduce blood glucose levels thus reducing complications from diabetes. This micronutrient may help ameliorate a diabetic condition!

Chromium enhances the body's sensitivity to insulin (a hormone that helps metabolize sugar). Chromium has been noted to reduce complications from diabetes by lowering blood glucose levels by 18% and glycosylated hemoglobin by 10%.

COENZYME Q10 (CoQ10): CoQ10 was discovered in 1957 by Fred Crane, M.D., from the University of Wisconsin. He isolated CoQ10 from beef hearts. CoQ10 is a Vitamin-like substance that resembles Vitamin E, which may be more powerful as an antioxidant. Of the 10 common coenzyme Qs, only CoQ10 is found in human tissue. CoQ10 declines with age and should be supplemented in the diet. CoQ10 plays a crucial role in the effectiveness of the immune system and the aging process!

The New England Institute reports that CoQ10 alone is effective in reducing mortality in experimental animals afflicted with tumors and leukemia. It's noted that CoQ10 may be helpful in the complete remission of many cancers!

In Japan, CoQ10 is being used in the treatment of heart disease, high blood pressure, and to enhance the immune system!

DIPHENYLHYDANTOIN (DPH): Trade name for DPH in the United States is Dilantin. Other trade names outside the United States are Aleviatan, Epamin, Epanutin, Eplin, and Idantoin. DPH's listed indication-of-use with the FDA is an anticonvulsant used effectively against epilepsy. Since the time this remarkable drug surfaced in 1938, physicians throughout the world have reported DPH useful for over 50 symptoms and disorders in over a hundred and fifty medical journals!

Almost everyone has heard of the Dreyfus Fund. Well, Jack Dreyfus is the author of a fascinating book concerning this amazing medication. Suffering from angry thoughts, depression, intense fear, and an overbusy brain occupied with emotions related to fear and anger for five years, Jack Dreyfus eventually linked one thing to another which led him to DPH.

ENZYMES: Enzymes are SO IMPORTANT for your health. Enzymes are ESSENTIAL for all chemical changes in your body. There are three types of enzymes:

- Metabolic enzymes which keeps your body functioning to its peak performance.
- Digestive enzymes in order to properly digest food.
- Food enzymes which are found in RAW FOOD! These enzymes also aid in proper food digestion. Enzymes are destroyed when food is cooked or heated above temperatures of 118 degrees.

Enzymes make minerals, proteins, Vitamins, and other components of our body work. Enzymes are vital to life and your performance. Every physical act from blinking, breathing, to walking can not take place without enzymes. Each year new enzymes are discovered and their amazing responsibilities they have with respect to your health. To date, thousands of enzymes have been discovered. For example, one very important enzyme is called Superoxide Dismutase (SOD). It's a super antioxidant and is working right now as you read this book! Without this enzyme, you would age very quickly! A 10-year old without SOD would look like a 70-year old person! Amazing huh!

FLAX SEED: In 1909, the average U.S. person consumed approximately 125 grams of fat per day. Today the average person in the U.S. consumes approximately 175 grams of fat, an increase of 40 percent or about 50 extra pounds per year and increasing! Of the total increase in the consumption of fats and oils, shortening, margarine, refined salad oil and cooking oils account for fifty percent. This increase in fat over the years is undoubtedly linked to the increase in degenerative diseases. In order to extend the shelf life of many products, essential fatty acids (good fat) have been purposely processed out of most foods. This is profitable for the manufacturer, but UNHEALTHY to the American consumer - YOU! Approximately 80% of Americans are deficient in essential fatty acids. Flax seed has a high content of essential fatty acids.

FOLIC ACID: Folic acid is considered brain food and needed for energy production and formation of red blood cells. It helps with protein metabolism. In addition to protecting against adult diseases, folic acid reduces the risk of birth defects in a fetus's developing nervous system by 50 percent.

The evidence is so strong that the Centers for Disease Control and Prevention (CDC) recommends that all women who may become pregnant consume 400mcg of folic acid a day.

Folic Acid helps regulate embryonic and fetal development of nerve cells vital for normal growth and development. Folic Acid works best with Vitamin B12.

A sore, red tongue may be one sign of Folic Acid deficiency. Significant sources of Folic Acid are barley, beans, beef, bran, brown rice, cheese, chicken, dates, green leafy vegetables, lamb, lentils, liver, milk, oranges, organ meats, split peas, pork, root vegetables, salmon, tuna, wheat germ, whole grains, whole wheat, and yeast.

In the United States alone, about 4,000 babies are born with neural tube birth defects (NTDs) each year (11 per day), which result from incomplete development of the brain (anencephaly) or spinal cord (spina bifida).

GLUCOSAMINE: Glucosamine is a natural occurring substance that is found in high concentrations in the joint structures of your body. Glucosamine's job is to stimulate the fabrication of cartilage components which are necessary for joint repair. As you grow older your body loses its ability to repair itself. Many people suffer from cartilage degradation, erosion, decrease or loss of joint movement, inflammation, and pain. The most common joints afflicted with osteoarthritis are the knees, hips, and fingers. Glucosamine Sulfate may be the answer if you suffer from osteoarthritis. Glucosamine Sulfate is noted to work on the cause of osteoarthritis. It addresses the root of the problem.

IRON: Iron is a mineral and is essential for life. Iron helps in body growth, prevents fatigue, and safeguards the body from disease. Iron is especially important to women more so than men. In one month women lose twice as much iron as men.
Follow the recommended dosage and instructions from the label and as per your doctor's instructions.

L-CARNITINE: L-Carnitine is noted to help strengthen the heart, lower blood fat levels, and relieve chest pains.
Follow the recommended dosage and instructions from the label and as per your doctor's instructions.

LECITHIN: Lecithin is any group of phosphatides found in all plant and animal tissues, produced commercially from egg yolks, soybeans, and corn. It's used in the processing of foods, pharmaceuticals, cosmetics, paints, inks, rubber, and plastics. Lecithin is a fat-like substance that is processed by the liver. Lecithin has important functions for your body. Lecithin is noted to be beneficial for the heart, memory, may help lower cholesterol level, and stimulate sexual vigor!

LIPOIC ACID: Most people and even doctors are not aware of lipoic acid (also known as alpha lipoic acid and thioctic acid) and its life-saving benefits. Lipoic acid is produced by your body and is a powerful antioxidant. It is both water soluble and fat soluble meaning it can access all parts of the cell to effectively fight free radicals! It also one of the most POWERFUL liver detoxifiers ever known!

Let me give you some background information on lipoic acid as a liver detoxifier: Approximately 20 years ago Burton Berkson, M.D., Ph.D, while a medical resident at Case Western Reserve Teaching Hospital Medical Center, was asked to treat 02 terminally ill from mushroom poisoning. One of the most deadliest poisons found in Mother Nature is called alpha amanitin and it's found the amanita mushroom. Eating the amanita mushroom causes irreversible liver destruction and death in 60% to 90% of cases! Dr. Berkson already had a Ph.D. in biology and his thesis was on mycology. Remembering an abstract on lipoic acid countering the killing effects of amanita poisoning, he called a friend at the National Institutes of Health who sent him some lipoic acid. Dr. Berkson then treated both patients with about 800mg administered in 4 infusions of 200mg. The lipoic acid COMPLETELY REVERSED THE LIVER DAMAGE IN BOTH PATIENTS! Both patients left the hospital in a few days! Lipoic acid has other therapeutic uses also.

MELATONIN: Melatonin is a natural hormone which is used as an organic alternative to sleeping aids and as a treatment for jet-lag. There have been 4,000 articles published on melatonin. Melatonin is inexpensive. It is a nonprescription supplement. According to my research, it has no toxic properties. Research indicates the following values of melatonin: a transducer, an overall governor of all energy functions, anti-aging, anti-arteriosclerotic, anti-infectious, anti-stress, anticarcinogenic, antitoxic, regulates endogenous opioid system, regulates hormone system, regulates immune system, regulates mineral metabolism, regulates oxidation reduction, and regulates respiration.

Swedish researchers Walter Pierpaoli and Georges Maestroni of the Institute of Integrative Bio-Medical Research in Locarno, Switzerland noted that when 10 healthy aging mice were given melatonin, their lifespan increased to 931 days, compared to 755 days for the control group. Not only did melatonin prolong their lifespan, but they also noted positive action on their performance and reversed or delayed symptoms of age-related debility, disease, and cosmetic decline!

MINERALS: Minerals are inorganic (do not contain carbon) dietary elements that are necessary for health. They are essential for strong bones and teeth, blood formation, and clotting. Minerals also help regulate body functions and fluid balance. Minerals are needed for proper composition of body fluids, formation of blood and bone, and maintenance of healthy nerve function. Minerals belong to two groups called macro (bulk) minerals and micro (trace) minerals. Bulk minerals are needed in larger amounts and include calcium, magnesium, sodium, potassium, and phosphorus. Trace minerals are required for good health and include chromium, copper, iodine, iron, manganese, selenium, and zinc. Read about some minerals, Vitamins, and other unknown super healthy supplements in Section 14.

PHYTOCHEMICALS: Phytochemicals are the natural chemical compounds found in all plants. Phytochemicals are naturally occurring chemicals in plants that give fruits, vegetables, grains, and legumes their medicinal, disease-preventing, health enhancing properties. Phytochemicals are noted to be powerful antioxidant nutrients.

Phytochemicals have recently demonstrated to scientists that they may be the newest weapon in the fight against disease. Initial evidence shows that phytochemicals may help encourage healthy blood pressure, support the immune system, assist the body in regulation of hormones, and may assist in mental and emotional health. The National Cancer Institute recently launched a multimillion dollar phytochemical research project. Synthetic forms of phytochemicals may be available years from now, but you can benefit from phytochemicals today by EATING THE RIGHT STUFF (fruits and vegetables) and adding quality supplements to your diet. At the time of this writing, scientists have discovered over 103,000 phytochemicals!

PROANTHOCYANIDINS: In the 1950's, Professor Jacques Masquelier of the University of Bordeaux, France isolated active components of the pine bark; they were found along the St. Lawrence River and other parts of the world.

There are 20,000 different types of and combinations of bioflavonoids. One particular group is vastly superior because it is water-soluble and highly bioavailable. This group of bioflavonoids is called proanthocyanidins!

The most powerful and health-enhancing and beneficial proanthocyanidins come from the bark of the maritime pine, Pinus maritima, growing along the southern coast of France from Bordeaux to the Spanish border. This bark contains the LARGEST AMOUNTS of the ACTIVE INGREDIENTS! Also called of Pycnogenol (PROANTHOCYANIDINS), these special compounds allow the Bordeaux pine to withstand the harsh winds of winter, the blinding sun and intense heat of summer, and the salty winds of the Atlantic Ocean!

ROYAL JELLY: Royal Jelly like bee pollen is packed with nutrients. Royal Jelly is the food that is fed ONLY to the Queen Bee in each hive! Royal Jelly is noted to increase the lifespan of the Queen bee 40 times longer than the average worker bee! Royal Jelly is noted to have a nutritious supply of 20 amino acids, minerals, Vitamins, and RNA-DNA factors. It's also known for its antibiotic effect. Nutrition Warehouse and BioEnergy Nutrients in Section 25 are just a couple of the companies that offer this nutritious food as well as bee pollen.

See Bee Pollen and Propolis in this section. How would you like the SUPER COMBINATION of Bee Pollen, Royal Jelly, and Propolis in one tablet form? I've come across a product called Super All Bee Power - Ultimate Energy Formula and it's manufactured by Y.S. Royal Jelly & Bee Farms, Sheridan, IL 60551. It also has Korean Ginseng and other ingredients in the product and it's Certified Organic!

SPIRULINA: The word Spirulina is derived from the latin word for *"helix"* or *"spiral"* for the physical configuration of the organism when it forms swirling, microscopic strands. Spirulina is a simple, single-celled algae that can be found in warm, alkaline bodies of fresh water. The nutrient content of algae meets the food needs of every cell of the higher organisms and makes it one of the most concentrated sources of pure food and nutrition in the universe. It's one of the great unharvested pastures of the world.

VANADYL SULFATEL Before I go into this amazing mineral, let me give you some information concerning diabetes. Most diabetics have too much insulin. Approximately 10% of diabetics have insufficient insulin production while the other 90% of diabetics are *"insulin resistant."* With this type of diabetes, your pancreas does its job by producing plenty of insulin - sometimes too much.

Even with plenty of insulin on hand it may not do its job because of your unhealthy diet, lack of exercise, or obesity... which may lead to being *"insulin resistant."* You now know how to possibly reverse being *"insulin resistant."* I highly suggest you go to Section 25 and see Dr. Julian Whitaker, Health & Healing, and order a book titled Reverse Diabetes. Anyway besides this very safe approach to help remedy your being *"insulin resistant,"* a mineral called vanadium which is a trace element, may turn things around for you! This amazing trace element is essential for cellular activity and the formation of bones & teeth and inhibits the formulation of cholesterol! In large doses, vanadyl sulfate (a form of vanadium) works like an oral insulin!

WATER: Yes, water (clean - uncontaminated) can make a difference in your health! Did you know your body is made up of 75% water? Your brain is made up of 85% water! We evolved from the ocean millions of years ago! Your body has close to the same proportioned salt content as ocean water! What am I getting at? If there is one immediate all-natural substance required for survival and good health besides air, it's water. Chronic dehydration may be linked to many diseases and pain!

In other words, just simply drinking more water and when to drink may ameliorate many common diseases! It's also been noted to help people lose weight! Drinking water is important and even more important is WHEN to drink it! Listen I could spend 3 or 4 pages discussing the importance of hydrating with water but I'll do one better. Below is a list of successful uses by simply drinking water and avoiding chronic dehydration!

- Allergies
- Asthma
- Chronic Fatigue Syndrome
- Colitis Pain
- Headache
- High Blood Cholesterol
- High Blood Pressure
- Low Back Pain
- Neck Pain
- Peptic Ulcer Disease
- Rheumatoid Arthritis
- Weight Loss

Drink plenty of pure - clean water (at least 10 to 12 eight-ounce glasses of water per day - more depending on your activity and the temperature and humidity readings) to prevent chronic dehydration!

WHOLE SALT: Table salt IS NOT Whole Salt, meaning it lacks over 80 minerals which protect the body from toxic effects of pure sodium chloride. Table salt (almost pure sodium chloride) is heated in an oven and stripped of its vital buffer minerals and may contribute to cardiovascular disease.

Everybody needs whole salt and not the refined salt you buy at the local grocery store. Whole salt is required for digestion, energy, regeneration of body cells, and many other biological functions of the body. Whole salt, used in moderation, is not only harmless but a valuable nutrient. One type of whole salt which contains over 80 buffer elements including magnesium is called Celtic Sea Salt. Celtic Sea Salt clean and unrefined, is hand-harvested in Brittany near the Celtic Sea in northwest France. Natural Celtic Sea Salt is obtained from the evaporation of the ocean's water. NO synthetic mineral supplement can equal the wealth of minerals that natural Celtic Seal Salt provides! Celtic Sea Salt is gathered after the ocean water is channeled daily into pristine ponds that is edged with natural waterways, wild grasses, and other green plants. The wind and sun evaporate the ocean water, leaving rich brine. Within hours, the crystals are gathered by hand.

SECTION 15 - Amazing Qualities And Benefits Of Aloe Vera!

Before I write anything about the amazing benefits of Aloe Vera, give me your undivided attention. DO NOT, I REPEAT, DO NOT go out and purchase any Aloe Vera at any store, health food store, or nutritional type stores. Why? According to experts, anyone, any company can put a few drops of Aloe Vera in a jug and call it *"100% Aloe Vera."* It should be illegal, but it isn't! Many of you that use Aloe products think you're using the good stuff that is packed with the beneficial active ingredients. Well, you're not! At the time of this writing (April 95), there are no quality control or federal laws regarding the label claims of many Aloe Vera products. I can personally vouch for one company that offers a bona fide authentic Aloe Vera product. I (author) have found and used their aloe vera products many times in the past with success. The name of this company is called LAMETCO. I'll tell you more about their authentic products on the following pages. First, let me tell you what a true aloe vera should have, should do and why it works!

Aloe Vera has many beneficial properties and many active chemicals and enzymes. The Aloe Vera plant was developed to survive in dry climates. The leaves are the very lifeblood of the plant itself and are large storehouses of nutrition and moisture. Herbal parts are taken from the whole leaf.

What is the healing secret of Aloe Vera?
An Aloe Vera leaf contains more than 99 percent water and less than 1 percent of active ingredients containing more than 200 nutritional substances. According to Ivan Danhof, Ph.D, M.D., Grand Prairie, Texas, the beneficial ingredients are several plant sugars produced in the leaf rind. These are called mucopolysaccharides; their trade name is acemannan. According to Medical world News (Dec. 1987), acemannan *"shows preliminary signs of boosting AIDS patients' immune systems and blocking the human immune-deficiency virus' spread, without toxic side effects."*

What are the benefits of the Amazing Aloe Vera plant?
There are over 200 different Aloe Vera species that grow around the world in dry regions. Aloe Vera is commonly used as a moisturizer, skin healer, and softener.

Aloe Vera is used on acne and blemishes, bruises, burns, cuts, eczema, insect stings, poison ivy, sun burns, ulcerated skin lesions, and welts. Aloe Vera is also known to aid in the healing of colitis, all colon problems, constipation, hemorrhoids, rectal itching, stomach disorders, and ulcers.

Many doctors describe the concentrate from Aloe Vera plant as a germ fighter, a pain killer, and an effective treatment for digestive and colon problems.

Lee Cowden, M.D., in Dallas, Texas, observed many benefits of from taking Aloe Vera (orally). Benefits include esophagitis, irritable bowel syndrome, lupus, mouth lesions, peptic ulcer, rheumatoid arthritis, osteoarthritis, sleep disturbances, sore throat, and ulcerative colitis.

In a six month study conducted by a family physician, 29 AIDS patients were given nutritional supplements, essential fatty acids, and Aloe Vera juice along with their regular diet. Most of the patients with symptoms reported their energy levels improved within 03 to 05 days and all began to gain weight!

Aloe Vera is a natural cleanser. It has the ability to penetrate through all layers of tissue and works as a local anesthetic to relieve pain on the skin surface and deep into tissue including joint and muscle pain. Aloe Vera is a bactericidal when it is maintained in high concentration for several hours in direct contact with bacteria. It is also a fungicidal and virucidal when in direct contact in high concentrations. It acts as a hemostatic agent to reduce bleeding. An antipyretic reducing the fever or heat of sores. It acts as an anti-inflammatory. It also acts as an antipruritic, stopping itching and burning (athletes feet, bee stings). Aloe Vera provides a wide range of amino acids, minerals, mucopolysaccharides, and mucoproteins. Mucopolysaccharides are important to bodily function. They protect each cell of the body against organisms such as bacteria, fungus, and virus. The body eliminates the production of mucopolysaccharides at puberty and must obtain them from food. Substantial amounts of mucopolysaccharides and mucoproteins are crustaceans and deep sea cold water fish. Aloe Vera dilates capillaries which increases blood supply.

SECTION 16 - Remarkable Benefits Of Colloidal Silver!

What is the history of Colloidal Silver?

Greeks and Romans utilized silver containers to keep liquids fresh. American settlers often put a silver dollar in milk to delay its spoiling and silver dollars were found in canteens to ensure the water was drinkable. In 1843 Seimi became the first researcher to systematically investigate colloids. In 1884 the German obstetrician F. Crede administered 1 percent silver nitrate to the eyes of newborn babies, virtually eliminating the incidence of disease causing blindness in newborn infants! Not until the late 1800's that Western scientists were able to prove what had already been known in Eastern medicine for thousands of years...that silver was a proven germ fighter!

Through the 1900's, Colloidal Silver gained rapid recognition as one of the best infection-preventive agents. This was short lived because the cost of silver and silver solutions could not be patented. New antibiotic drugs were the choice of medical treatment. After 30 years of antibiotic drugs, many types of bacteria built an immunity to their action. The comeback of silver in medicine began in the 1970's. In March 28, 1994 issue of Newsweek Magazine devoted six full pages to this subject. The large bold type words on the front cover declared, *"ANTIBIOTICS...The End of Miracle Drugs?......WARNING: NO LONGER EFFECTIVE AGAINST KILLER BUGS.... In 1992, 13,300 hospital patients died of infections that resisted every drug doctors tried."* The timely re-emergence of Colloidal Silver may prove to be one of the most powerful remedies to offset some of the serious problems we now face.

What is a Colloid?

A colloid is a substance that is composed of particles which are very small but larger than molecules. These particles in a colloid don't dissolve but remain suspended in a suitable liquid. Did you know all living things exist in a colloidal state? Your body can more readily use medications that are already in a colloidal state versus many over-the-counter medications which are in a crystalline state which your body converts to a colloidal state.

What is Colloidal Silver?

Colloidal Silver is pure electrically charged particles of silver that are 0.01 to about 0.001 microns in diameter and suspended in distilled water. According to medical literature, the best quality of Colloidal Silver is actually gold in color and has the quality for injection use.

What is the therapeutic value of Colloidal Silver?

According to medical journals from around the world, therapeutic value of Colloidal Silver is annotated as a POWERFUL wide-spectrum antibiotic that disables the enzyme that all one-celled bacteria, fungi, and viruses use for their oxygen metabolism causing them to SUFFOCATE in six minutes or less upon contact which was recently tested at UCLA Medical Labs!

The majority of prescription antibiotics kill only a few different disease-causing organisms. Colloidal Silver is noted to be successful against **650 plus disease organisms** without causing any known side-effects! Colloidal Silver is non-irritating to tissue - no toxicity! Colloidal Silver can be used to disinfect, or better yet support, your immune system. However, Colloidal Silver does not kill or inhibit all forms of bacteria, virus, or fungus. Some essential bacteria is necessary to maintain life!

How do I use Colloidal Silver?

Depending on the problem, Colloidal Silver is tasteless and can be taken orally for a wide variety of conditions such as candida, chronic fatigue, parasites, shingles, staph, strep, and over 600 viral and bacterial diseases. Colloidal Silver has been noted to be successful used in septic conditions of the mouth including pyorrhea and tonsillitis. When applied to the skin, Colloidal Silver can help with troublesome acne, athlete's foot, open sores, and warts. Colloidal Silver can be applied to the eyes to help conjunctivitis as well as other forms of inflammation and infection of the eyes with no stinging or irritation. Colloidal Silver can also be used anally, vaginally, and atomized into the lungs and nose. It can also be used in injectable form in 100cc bottles for qualified health professionals.

SECTION 17 - Unbelievable Benefits Of Essiac\Flor*Essence!

First of all, let me give you some historical information concerning this very beneficial and all natural formula! The formula that we'll talk about in this section was originally made by native Canadians in Northern Ontario. In 1922 a former cancer patient told nurse named Rene Caisse about a herbal tea that had cured her breast cancer! Rene Caisse took sincere interest in this herbal formula and began to share it. When Rene Caisse's aunt recovered from inoperable cancer after taking this herbal tea, doctors began to refer their hopeless cases to Rene Caisse. Rene Caisse and Dr. Fisher conducted many experiments and they finally refined this herbal tea and named it Essiac (Caisse spelled backwards). The following eight years Rene Caisse ran a clinic in Bracebridge, Ontario.

Nurse Caisse came under many threats of arrest by authorities for practicing medicine without a license. Nurse Caisse charged no fees at her clinic in Bracebridge, Ontario so she was financially unable to defend herself in court. The Essiac tea was not scientifically proven to work and she was not a doctor. Doctors and former patients supported and campaigned for Rene's exemption. After the threats of arrest, fines, and jail, Rene Caisse decided to close the clinic. However, her herbal formula Essiac had already proven itself to many of Rene's patients!

Over 55,000 people (former patients and their families and friends), including several leading doctors, petitioned the Ontario Government to allow Caisse (Essiac) *"administer the remedy... without the threat of interference from authorities."*

THOUSANDS of people in Canada suffering from terminal cancer have been successfully treated and reportedly many cured with this herbal remedy!

President Kennedy's personal physician, Charles A. Brusch, M.D., helped perfect the original Essiac formula and cured himself of deadly bowel cancer! Dr. Brusch worked with the Presidential Cancer Commission, the American Cancer Society, and the National Cancer Institute. After 10 years of research, Dr. Brusch presented his findings, *"Essiac is a cure for cancer, period. All studies done at laboratories in the United States and Canada support this conclusion."*

Upon this conclusion from Dr. Brusch, the federal government issued a gag order and said *"You got one of two choices, either you keep quiet about this or we'll haul you off to military prison and you'll never be heard of again."*

People from around the world have anxiously travelled to Canada to get their hands on what reportedly could be the most effective non-toxic remedy AGAINST CANCER!

Essiac is an incredibly effective Canadian Herbal Cancer Remedy which has, for more than 50 years, successfully treated thousands of people suffering from various forms of terminal cancer! Few promising treatments, if any, can offer such enormous hope to cancer sufferers.

The original formula was called Essiac which was named after Rene Caisse spelled backwards. Another formula with four additional herbs is called Flor*Essence. Go to your local library and not only read about the historical information concerning Rene Caisse's amazing find, but also the carefully documented healing facts and testimonials in The Essiac Report, by Richard Thomas!

When referring to Essiac, Essiac and Flor*Essence are the same herbal formulation except Flor*Essence has four additional herbs.

What is ESSIAC\Flor*Essence?
Essiac is a non-toxic combination of four herbs that are perfectly proportioned in such a way that their separate beneficial effects are synergistically enhanced. Essiac is made from organically grown herbs harvested at the peak of ripeness and free of toxic herbicides, pesticides, and chemical fertilizers. Essiac herbs are grown in accordance with European Standards (highest quality control standards in the world). Essiac herbs pass 02 microbiological assays before blending and after blending. The Essiac herbs are finally assayed by High Performance Liquid Chromatography to ensure the identity and purity of the materials. Essiac is non-toxic and drug free, powerful immune system therapy, and an effective herbal remedy.

SECTION 18 - Super Health With Super Blue Green Algae (SBGA)!

What is Super Blue Green Algae (SBGA)?

Algae are among this planet's most ancient organisms that are found in every rich soil in every body of water. From the most largest and vast oceans to the tiniest puddles of water in the hottest springs to the coldest streams. Algae is responsible 90% of the world's photosynthesis, consuming carbon dioxide and producing oxygen and food for the entire food chain. Without this nutritious algae there would be no life in the seas and very little on land!

Algae has been consumed by man for hundreds of years. Only recently has algae been praised by scientists as the group of high protein-containing organisms which are the most likely to provide man with sufficient amounts of nutrients for the future.

Previously, the best known species of blue green algae available for human consumption were spirulina and chlorella. Both spirulina and chlorella are grown artificially in man-made ponds and fed whatever man has decided that their proper nutrition should be.

Is Super Blue Green Algae superior to Spirulina and Chlorella products?

Aphanizomenon flos-aquae, better known as Super Blue Green Algae, is a completely wild algae living in Upper Klamath Lake located in Southern Oregon far from the pollution of the cities, their sewage, and far from industrial and agricultural activities (pesticides and herbicides). Upper Klamath Lake is fed by 17 volcanic mountain streams and rivers shaping this high desert lake into an actual nutrient trap! Klamath Lake is protected by the high Cascade Mountains and fed by geothermal hot springs and 4000 square miles of melting snow. All the minerals your body needs are contained here in the basin - in chelated form - to become food for the micro algae. Super Blue Green Algae has a complete balance of Vitamins, except for Vitamin D (sunlight) and Vitamin E (the algae's high chlorophyll contents help produce Vitamin E naturally in the body). It is rich in the B Vitamins, including B-12, and it has the highest known source of chlorophyll, which is 300% higher than alfalfa!

Blue Green Algae at Klamath Lake grows during the summer months. The Blue Green Algae is harvested fresh from the lake on a daily basis and flash frozen to preserve its vital nutrients. The nutrient rich soils of the Cascade Range support the enormous photosynthetic environment that IS NOT DUPLICATED ANYWHERE ELSE IN THE WORLD.

SECTION 19 - Super Healing Herbs And Plants!

Before we get into the super healing benefits of herbs let me tell you why herbs and all alternative medicine I'm telling you about throughout this book is unfairly ridiculed.

Natural and inexpensive alternative treatments cannot be patented to generate big profits because they're simply natural, which means these alternative treatments are of no high value to conventional health-care where billions and billions of dollars are being made each year. Health-care in the United States runs more than a trillion dollars a year! So, if your doctor or someone you know scoffs at alternative medicine, let them read this book. You might convert your friend and even that stubborn doctor! OK, let me tell you about Super Healing Herbs And Plants!

Modern medicine is taking a second look at herbal remedies and realizing that herbs aren't just for flavoring, but have medicinal qualities! The earliest example of herbal medicine dates to the third century B.C., *"History of Plants"* by a greek scholar named Theophrastus. A second century A.D. healer named Dioscorides was a physician to Roman Armies. Dioscorides wrote large numbers of works on herbal remedies and was the unchallenged authority of herbs for centuries throughout Europe. During the Middle Ages, monks became involved in herbal medicine. Monastery herb gardens were cultivated to benefit the sick and suffering who went there for remedies and cures. Village dwellers gathered herbs from their cultivated gardens or from the roadside. They prepared concoctions, infusions, and salves to treat a variety of diseases and illnesses.

Alfalfa -- Herbal parts are taken from its leaves, petals, flowers, and sprouts. Alfalfa provides biotin, calcium, choline, inositol, iron, magnesium, PABA (para-aminobenzoic acid), phosphorus, potassium, protein, sodium, sulfur, tryptophan (amino acid), Vitamins A, B complex, C, D, E, K, and U. Alfalfa alkalizes and detoxifies the body especially in the liver. Alfalfa is beneficial for anemia, all colon disorders, arthritis, diabetes, hemorrhaging, promoting pituitary gland function, and helps remedy ulcers. Alfalfa also contains an antifungus agent.

Bilberry -- During World War II, English Air Force pilots and navigators consumed bilberry preserves to nourish their eyes and aid in night vision! At the present, there have been over 70 clinical studies conducted with Bilberry and have demonstrated that this exceptional extract may help combat visual fatigue and aid eyes' adaptation to darkness. Extensive studies have confirmed that Bilberry, Vaccinium myrtillus, helps support the small capillaries that feed eye muscles and nerves, which may inhibit the damage caused by blood vessel deterioration.

Blessed Thistle -- Herbal parts are taken from various parts. Blessed Thistle provides cincin and volatile oils. It is noted for increasing appetite, helps heal the liver, aids in the flow of breast milk in a nursing mother, improves circulation, purifies the blood, strengthens the heart, and alleviates pneumonitis (inflammation of lung tissue). Blessed Thistle could be used as brain food!

Follow the recommended dosage and instructions from the label and as per your doctor's instructions.

Capsicum (cayenne) -- Herbal parts are taken from berries and fruits. It acts as a catalyst for herbs and provides apsaicine, capsacutin, capsaicin, capsanthine, capsico, PABA, Vitamins A, B1, B2, B3, B5, B6, B9, C (rich source), E, ascorbic acid, calcium, dihydrocapsaicin, homocapsaicin, homodihydrocapsaicin, iron, magnesium, phosphorus, potassium, selenium, sulphur, and zinc. Capsicum is the source of over 100 varieties of Cayenne Pepper, from heat ranges of mild paprika to the extremely hot habanera. It's been used for medicinal purposes for thousands of years! Capsicum aids digestion, improves circulation, and stops bleeding from ulcers. It is noted to also be good for the kidneys, lungs, spleen, pancreas, heart, and stomach.

Chaparral -- This amazing herb is native to the American southwest. Native Americans in that area have used chaparral for centuries! Chaparral is one of the world's oldest plants. No wonder chaparral is noted to have POWERFUL antioxidant properties! Its herbal parts are taken from its waxy leaves. Native American Indians (Apache, Hopi, Navajo, and Pima) used and knew this medicinal plant to *"be good for everything."*

Acting as free radical scavenger, chaparral helps protect you against harmful effects of radiation and sun exposure. Chaparral helps with arthritis, leg cramps, pain relief, purify the blood, and skin disorders. Chaparral helps protect against formation of tumors and cancer cells. It is also noted to help improve kidney, liver, and lung function.

Chlorella -- Chlorella is noted to be a natural medicinal algae. Chlorella has more chlorophyll and DNA\RNA than any known edible food. It has more protein than beef or soybeans, generous amounts of B-12, more nucleic acid than sardines, a great source of beta carotene, 19 amino acids, and more than 20 Vitamins and minerals!

More than 800 scientific medical journal articles have established Chlorella as totally non-toxic!

The Hippocrates Institute in West Palm Beach, Florida has effectively treated 1,000 patients with Chlorella who endured blood sugar problems, heart disease, liver disorders, Pancreas disorders, and other ailments!

SECTION 20 - Healing Power Of Chelation Therapy!

What is Chelation Therapy?

American Board of Chelation Therapy (ABCT) defines chelation therapy as *"A form of medical therapy designed to restore cellular homeostasis by the use of metal binding and/or bio-inorganic agents. The proper application of this modality also requires knowledge of nutrition and exercise, as well as expertise in helping to implement other lifestyle changes."* The chelation process originated in 1893 with a French - Swiss chemist named Alfred Werner who received the Nobel Prize in 1913 for his pioneering work.

Chelation Therapy uses EDTA (Ethylene Diamine Tetraacetic Acid) or other supplements that carry out heavy metals like lead, cadmium, and arsenic as well as other foreign substances from the body. In the process of chelation, a larger protein molecule surrounds or encloses a mineral atom. The purpose of chelation is to increase the flow of blood to the vital organs and tissues of the body by reducing calcium deposits in the arteries and blood vessels. Chelation agents are used to bind with heavy toxic metals such as cadmium, lead, and mercury to excrete them from the body.

Chelation Therapy works like a magnet attracting metal shavings! When administered as an infusion into the blood stream, it removes metals and metal compounds from the body including but not limited to, calcium (works against calcium in atherosclerotic pathology). Most people are unaware that Chelation Therapy exists and has been documented and proven to rejuvenate the arteries and renew blood flow throughout the body WITHOUT SURGERY! That vital blood flow is instrumental in many healing qualities of this amazing therapy! KEEP READING!

Is Chelation Therapy considered nutritional therapy?

Chelation Therapy helps vital nutrients like carbohydrates, enzymes, fats, hormones, minerals, proteins, Vitamins, and other food substances complete their metabolic actions in your body. These nutrients also help detoxify your body. Chelation Therapy helps increase the amount of needed oxygen used at the CELLULAR LEVEL!

Over 75 trillion cells in your body need oxygen among other elements to function, thus HEALING AT THE CELLULAR LEVEL instead of treating symptoms with drugs! Again, each one of those 75 trillion cells need oxygen to function properly. Chelation Therapy can remove plaque from 75,000 miles of blood vessels throughout your entire body! Chelation Therapy assists the oxygenation process and significantly affects your health and health-related problems for the better. Especially those health-related problems involving the cardiovascular system, nerves, and sex organs.

Chelation Therapy, both intravenous and oral, helps prevent or overcome six of the 11 big killer diseases of Americans which are: heart disease, cancer, infectious diseases, diabetes, stroke, accidents, pneumonia, cirrhosis of the liver, arteriosclerosis, suicides, and infant death! Except for infant death, suicide, pneumonia, and accidents, Chelation Therapy prevents or reverses the top killers of Americans.

Can Chelation Therapy be considered to avoid amputation?
It is noted that many patients that had exhausted all traditional forms of treatment for endstage occlusive peripheral arterial disease were referred to peripheral vascular surgeons for amputation of their gangrenous limb. Patients turned to certified Chelation Therapists. Chelation Therapy (EDTA) was therapeutic in reversing ischemia (cessation of the flow of blood because of a blocked artery). If you or anyone you know is faced with possible amputation of a limb, LOOK into Chelation Therapy. See a Certified Chelation Therapist in your area for professional advice on this and many other health-related concerns. Read on for referrals!

What types of degenerative diseases can Chelation Therapy ameliorate, control, reverse, prevent, or at least ease the symptoms?
Below is a partial list of common degenerative diseases:

- Alzheimer's Disease
- Arteriosclerosis
- Arthritis
- Cancer
- Cataracts
- Cirrhosis
- Diabetes
- Diabetic Retinopathy
- Gangrene

SECTION 21 - Common Health Concerns And Healthy Information You Should Know!

ACNE: Acne is a skin inflammatory disease caused by an overproduction of sebum which is a fatty secretion produced by small glands under the skin, causing clogging of the pores and may lead to a bacterial infection. Changing to a healthier diet by eliminating alcohol, saturated fats, soft drinks, sugars, and smoking may reduce acne. Beta carotene A (healthy skin Vitamin) 25,000IU four times a day, Zinc picolinate (stimulates antibodies to avoid infectious bacteria on the skin) 50mg two times a day, and Vitamin C (ester C) 1000mg four times a day may remedy the acne problem. Herbs like Horsetail tone the skin and Red Clover purifies and cleanses the skin and helps the liver remove toxins from the body. Dandelion and Jojoba are liver cleansers. L-Cysteine, 500mg twice daily on an empty stomach, acts like an antioxidant for the skin. Apply Aloe Vera three times a day.

AGING: Aging is a degenerative process of the breakdown of cellular matter. People are living longer but may enjoy it less. 100 years ago, 01 in 10 reached the age of 65. Most of those that did, had been worn out by lack of proper nutrition, disease, and backbreaking physical labor.

How old you are doesn't depend on your chronological age, but your Biological age (your body's age in terms of critical life signs & cellular process) and Psychological age (how old you feel). Aging may be reversible!

Tufts University researchers discovered that muscle mass, a key to the body's overall vitality, doesn't decline with age. Twelve men aged 60-72 on a three month weight training program, could lift heavier boxes than the 25 year old workers in the lab. Milder weight training programs proved equally successful for people over 95!

The Tufts University researchers found that regular physical exercise also reverses the following typical effects of biological ageing: excess body fat, low blood-sugar tolerance, high blood pressure, high cholesterol/HDL ratio, low metabolic rate, poor body temperature regulation, reduced aerobic capacity, reduced bone density, and reduced strength.

According to researchers at Tufts University, a group of 90-year-old men and women increased their strength by an amazing average of 174 percent after only eight weeks (03 sessions per week) on weight machines.

A study in Southern California found that the longest-lived followed the following simple rules:

- Avoid eating between meals
- Avoid smoking
- Drink moderately
- Eat breakfast
- Not significantly overweight or underweight
- Regular physical activity
- Sleep 07 to 08 hours

ALZHEIMER'S DISEASE: A ultimately fatal illness, Alzheimer's disease first destroys mental functioning including memory, speech, comprehension, and awareness. Almost 50% of all Americans have it by age 85. The incidence of Alzheimer's disease in the United States today is more than 02.5 million, afflicting approximately 15 percent of Americans over the age of sixty-five.

Acetylcarnitine is a natural substance produced by your body. According to a clinical test at the Mario Negri Institute for Pharmacological Research in Milan, Italy acetylcarnitine taken orally significantly improved attention span, memory, verbal capacity and other mental functioning in 130 Alzheimer's patients. Throughout the United States, 27 centers are in their final stages (if they haven't already been completed) of human trials using acetylcarnitine. Food & Drug Administration approval is near at hand if it hasn't already been approved at the time of this writing.

DMSO has demonstrated promising relief to those suffering from arthritis. DMSO is also noted as a potent free radical scavenger, helps improve short-term memory in Alzheimer's patients, and benefits those patients afflicted with scleroderma and Raynaud's. DMSO is very safe and can be administered intramuscularly by injection, intravenously, orally, and topically on the skin.

IMMUNE SYSTEM: The immune system is a combination of cells and proteins that assist in the host's ability to fight and resist foreign substances such as viruses and harmful bacteria. The liver, spleen, thymus, bone marrow, and lymphatic system are interrelated in the immune system's normal function.

A Florida investigator, Tarig Abdullah, M.D., at the Akbar Clinic and Research Center in Panama, Florida found that raw garlic could dynamically heighten the powers of the immune systems natural killer cells (first line of defence against infectious diseases), including cancer.

In a study, Dr. Abdullah himself ate 12 to 15 cloves of garlic a day. A control group took garlic supplements and the third group took nothing. The natural killer cells from the different bloods (test groups) were combined with cancer cells.

The killer cells taken from the blood of those taking garlic supplements (control group) and eating garlic (Dr. Abdullah) DESTROYED 140 to 160 PERCENT MORE CANCER than the third group that didn't eat any garlic at all! According to Dr. Abdullah's report, the discovery has far reached implications not only for cancer and infections, but also for AIDS. Garlic may boost the ability to overcome the many fungal-type infections that hit AIDS patients. Dr. Abdullah brags that he eats several raw garlic cloves every single day and HAS NOT HAD A SINGLE COLD since initiating the garlic regimen in 1973!

Refined sugar (cane and beet) has been linked to impairing the immune functioning system. Studies have shown that sugar can distort the chemistry of antibodies or reduce lymphocyte cells which are important to the immune system.

According to Dr. Elaine Fox (The Guide to a Healthier Diet -- Eat Well\Be Well video), sugar affects the effectiveness of your body's immune system by the way white blood cells are able to fight foreign invaders.

In Japan, Coenzyme Q10 (CoQ10) is being used in the treatment of heart disease, high blood pressure, and to enhance the immune system.

The herbs aloe vera, echinacea, and barley greens are noted for their immune booster capabilities. Read about these healing herbs in Section 19!

Shark cartilage has only three years (as of Oct. 1995) of research while bovine cartilage has more than 40-years and $7 million in scientific backing. Bovine cartilage has been successfully used in treatment of cancer for more than 20 years! It is also effective against rheumatism and arthritic diseases, immunological skin disorders, and herpes infections.

SECTION 22 - 60+ Amazing Health Enhancing Alternative Medicine Practices That Work!

(the full section is included in the FULL VERSION)

In 1992, the National Institutes of Health established an Office of Alternative Medicine to provide grants to test if the mounting plethora of natural medical remedies really work. The King County Council in Washington state plans to establish the very first government-subsidized natural medicine clinic. The clinic will be staffed by naturopaths offering dietary supplements of enzymes & Vitamins, acupuncture, botanical fluids, and much more!

You must be aware of alternative medicine practices. Why? In 1990, why did 425,000,000 Americans visit providers of unconventional (alternative) therapy? You must see Alternative Medicine Yellow Pages and Future Medicine Publishing Company in Section 25 for THOUSANDS of sources of Alternative Medicine and valuable information.

Acupressure & Oriental Body Therapy -- Acupressure uses the pressure of the fingers and hands. Acupuncture uses needles. Acupressure is the older of the two techniques. It is an effective self-care and prevention health care treatment for tension-related ailments. Oriental bodywork developed primarily through a combination of instinct and hands-on experience. Its principles and healing techniques integrate breathing, meditations, herbal remedies, and massage.

Alexander Technique -- Frederick Matthias Alexander pioneered an effective approach to rebalancing the body through awareness, movement, and touch. Alexander was aware that the correct relationship of one's head, neck. and back is essential for proper movement and functioning. Poor use of the body can contribute to many diseases including arthritis, debilitating curvatures of the spine, rheumatism, and a variety of gastrointestinal and breathing disorders. Over 2,500 people worldwide have been trained in the Alexander Technique. Alexander technique has enhanced the performance of people associated with dance, drama, music, and speech. Athletes have found that the Alexander Technique enhanced their performance as well as relieved chronic pain.

Amma Therapy -- Amma Massage is based on ancient Oriental traditions that gave birth to Shiatsu and Kahuna energy-based massage. Amma works *"tsubos,"* or energy points, stroking away from the heart.

Applied Kinesiology -- Applied Kinesiology consists of testing various muscle and nerve reflexes in the body to determine the strength or weakness of various organ systems. Applied Kinesiology can also be used to determine the receptivity of the body to various remedies thereby aiding in restoring health.

Aromatherapy -- Aromatherapy is the science of utilizing essential oils from botanical sources with anti-viral and anti-fungal properties for the treatment of a variety of maladies. The selected essential oils can be inhaled and in some cases ingested. In France, aromatherapy is used in hospitals. Many aspects of aromatherapy make it a valuable system self-care.

Aston-Pattering -- Aston-Pattering consists of an integrated system of environmental modifications, fitness training, movement education and 3-D soft tissue work.

Auricular Therapy -- It is also called Auriculotherapy. Auricular Therapy, or ear acupuncture, is a sophisticated treatment using an electronic instrument called Stim Flex. The Stim Flex stimulates specific points on the ear with undetectable microcurrents. Auricular Therapy is pain-free and no puncture is involved.

This therapy is noted to relieve pain, all kinds of pain. in minutes! It is noted to have other amazing benefits like reversing stroke symptoms!

Autogenic Training and Therapy -- Autogenic Training (AT) is a systematized series of attention-focusing exercises designed to generate a state of mind and body relaxation. Autogenics is similar to self-hypnosis and is used to gain deep relaxation and enhance one's recuperative and self-healing powers. Autogenic means self-generated. AT's aim is to give trainees the skills to put themselves in a relaxed state without depending on a trainer or guide. Autogenics assume a deep faith in the brain's and body's own ability to regulate itself!

Ayurvedic Medicine -- Ayurvedic Medicine is an ancient system of medicine from India. It is based on treating patients according to three metabolic types. Ayurvedic medicine places great value on detoxification, diet, exercise, herbal medicine, and meditation. Ayurvedic medicine is effective in treating a wide range of chronic conditions.

SECTION 23 - Health Care Titles and Abbreviations!

Audiologist -- Specialist in hearing disorders.

Cardiologist -- A heart specialist.

Chiropractor -- The core or foundation of chiropractic's approach is the relationship between the spinal column\musculoskeletal structures of the body and the nervous system. When misalignments (subluxations) in the spine occur, they may cause nerve interference. These interruptions cause pain and lower body defenses. Removing misalignments and restoring normal nerve function optimizes the body's inherent ability to heal itself.

Clinical Psychologist (Ph.D.) -- Psychologists are called doctors because they have a doctoral degree in psychology. Psychologists are not medical doctors. They counsel people with mental and emotional problems. Some clinical psychologists that have a master's degree work with patients, but do not use the title *"Doctor."*

Dermatologist -- A skin specialist.

Eye Care Ophthalmologist (M.D.) -- Ophthalmologists are D.O.'s or M.D.'s. They specialize in the diagnosis and treatment of diseases of the eye. They prescribe eyeglasses and contact lenses as well as prescribe drugs and perform surgery. They treat patients who have cataracts and glaucoma.

Family Practitioner (M.D.) -- They are M.D.'s or D.O.'s who specialize in providing comprehensive (complete care with aid of specialist if necessary) health care for all family members, on a continuing basis, regardless of age or sex.

Gastroenterologist -- A specialist in disease of the digestive tract.

General Care, M.D. -- General Care, Doctors of Medicine, using all accepted treatments of medical care. M.D.'s complete medical school plus three to seven years of graduate medical education. Must be licensed by the state in which they practice. These doctors treat diseases and injuries, do checkups, prescribe drugs, preventive care, and do some surgery.

SECTION 24 – Stress And The Money Connection!

OK, let's get started with this section.

Stress is a physical or psychological stimulus which, when impinging upon an individual, produces strain or disequilibrium.

Emotional stress can cause arteries to constrict throughout your body. When this occurs in the heart, it is called coronary heart spasm.

Put yourself in the following situation and put aside faith in your religion and love from family and friends.

- Your life is dictated by your job, its scheduled hours, your set salary, and the time and amount of time allotted for a vacation.

- Supporting yourself and your family requires huge amounts of money! You need large amounts of money for loans, the use of credit cards to acquire the necessities of life (house, clothes, car, food, education, and insurance) in a timely manner, which in turn controls how you spend your future income from your job.

- Your job may be at jeopardy due to politics, economy, and health which brings stress simply pondering the thought of losing your job. There are so many long term and short term debts to pay in order to keep you and your family content. Even if you were guaranteed a job till you're 65 or so, you're still in debt and always will be due to your set salary and those ever nagging long-term and short-term debts, nor are you in control of your life.

- You now lose your job and stress like no other has hit you from all sides. Your family is depending on you. All long-term and short-term debts are snowballing and the unthinkable - the thought of being homeless has now entered your overstressed mind.

Folks the scenario you just read in part or whole is absolutely real for most of the people living within the United States! No, it's not as bad as Third World countries, but the stress accompanying your daily lives can be greatly reduced if you could control how you want to live and where you want to live as well as establish your own lifestyle (your hopes and wishes become real). You can't possibly do that without money and a great deal of it.

SECTION 25 - Points Of Contact (1,500+ - full version) And Phone Numbers For Your Health, Safety, Save Money, Make Money, And Peace Of Mind!

In this section you'll discover no less than 1,500 government agencies, organizations, and private companies that are in the business of providing information and products with respect to your health, safety, help you save money, make you money, and for your peace of mind! You'll discover many healthy products and information that is defying medical science! You'll have access to information that will enhance your overall health, safety, and peace of mind! In this section, as well as this entire book, you'll soon discover that INFORMATION IS YOUR BEST AND MOST LOYAL FRIEND!

Keep in mind that this section may already be out-of-date due to area code changes, address changes, phone number changes, company or agency name changes. If you find an error in any Point of Contact, write to IRIS (Intensive Research Information Services in this section) and I'll gladly update this section for new clients. PLEASE TAKE ADVANTAGE of this section and call or write as many Points of Contact as you wish according to your concern and even your curiosity. Toll-free numbers may be 800 or 888.

ABC NEWS
Videos---1-800-913-3434
Transcripts---1-800-All-NEWS
ABC News on Demand on American On Line-----------------------------1-800-772-4222
ABC Audience Relations and Comments----------------------------------1-212-456-7477
ABC NEWS offers a variety of videos and transcripts with respect to public health. Call the numbers above and request information.

Academy for Guided Imagery, The--1-800-726-2070
The Academy for Guided Imagery, P.O. Box 2070, Mill Valley, CA 94942. Call and ask for free information or talk to one of their representatives Monday through Thursday from 9 a.m. to 4 p.m., Pacific Standard Time. You'll receive three brochures on their amazing products. See Guided Imagery in Section 22.

Wyoming Health Insurance Pool--------------------------------1-800-442-2764
Wyoming Health Insurance Pool, P.O. Box 2256, Cheyenne, WY 82003. Health Insurance
Coverage for the Hard-to-Insure. Offers comprehensive health insurance to state residents with
serious medical conditions who can't find a company to insure them.

Xenejenex--1-800-228-2495
Xenejenex, 29 Sawyer Road, Waltham, Massachusetts 02154. Call Xenejenex for their free
product catalog. You'll receive a 10-page color brochure and order form on their video products.
Main titles include Women's Health Set (4 videos), Exercise\Cardiac Rehabilitation Set (5
videos), Wellness Set (7 videos), and Health Specific Set (5 videos).

Zand--1-310-822-0500
McZand Herbal, Inc., P.O. Box 5312, Santa Monica, CA 90409. Zand offers a variety of herbal
formulas like Active Herb for stress, energy, and performance; Herbal Programs for the Winter;
and Herbal Formulas for Women's Health. All these are comprised of dozens and dozens of
herbs that are already prepared in liquid, capsule, tablet, and powder form. Zand also offers
herbalozenges for cold symptom relief! Call or write for free information. They'll send you
colorful and informative brochures.

SECTION 26 – Glossary Of Doctor Words And Other Information You Should Know!

Abscess -- An abscess is an inflamed or swollen area of the body tissue in which pus gathers.

Abstract -- A statement summarizing the important points of a given text.

Absorption -- Absorption is the process by which nutrients are absorbed through the intestinal tract into the bloodstream to be used by the body. If the nutrients aren't absorbed, the body becomes deficient in building and healing substances.

Agoraphobia -- Agoraphobia is the fear of leaving home for fear of a panic disorder attack in a public place, or while driving.

AIDS -- AIDS stands for Acquired Immuno Deficiency Syndrome, a condition in which the immune system cells have been infected with the human immunodeficiency virus. The body can no longer fight off illnesses caused by bacteria, fungus, virus, or other pathogens because the compromised immune system is unable to defend it. AIDS compromises the competency of the immune system and is characterized by persistent lymphadenopathy and various opportunistic infections such as Pneumocystis carnipneumonia, cytomegalovirus, disseminated histoplasmosis, candidiasis and isosporiasis, and malignancies such as Kaposi's sarcoma; the etiologic agent is HTLV-III, transmissible by blood fluids such as blood and semen. Early symptoms include diarrhea, fatigue, fever, headache, heavily coated white tongue, lung infection, night sweat, swollen lymph glands, and weight loss.

Alcohol -- Alcohol is a drug. Like sedatives, alcohol depresses the central nervous system and is the major psychoactive ingredient in wine, beer, and distilled liquors.

Alcoholism -- Alcoholism is alcohol abuse, dependence or addiction, chronic heavy drinking, or intoxication resulting in impairment of health, dependency as a coping mechanism, and increased adaptation to the effects of alcohol requiring increasing doses to achieve and sustain a desired effect.

Alkaloid(s) -- One of a group of organic alkaline substances obtained from plants. Alkaloids react with acids to form salts that are used for medical purposes.

All Bran -- See bran in this section.

Allergy -- An allergy is an immunologic response (inappropriate or harmful) to substances like drugs, foods, infectious agents, inhalants, pollen, or other contaminations. These substances are harmless to most people. Conventional treatment like antihistamines, cortisone, decongestants and desensitizing injections are established therapies.

Allicin -- Allicin is the active ingredients in garlic. Allicin is a bacteriostasis, meaning it inhibits further growth of bacteria. Read the very health enhancing beneficial effects of garlic in Section 13.

Alloy -- A combination of two or more metals. See mercury in Section 11.

Aloe Vera -- SEE Aloe Vera in Section 15!

Alternative Medicine -- Alternative Medicine is different from established conventional medicine. See Section 22 for more than 60 Alternative Medicine Practices that really work!

Aluminum Toxicity -- Foods cooked in aluminum produce chloride poison, neutralize the digestive juices, and produce acidosis and ulcers. Unwanted aluminum is deposited in the brain and nervous system tissues. Excessive amounts of aluminum are linked to Alzheimer's disease. Aluminum is also found in many consumable products.

Alzheimer's Disease -- Alzheimer's is a degenerative disease of the brain, often occurring in middle age, causing progressive loss of mental faculties. It is also called *"presenile dementia,"* previously classified as senile dementia. Alzheimer's disease is characterized by tangled nerve fibers surrounding the hippocampus. When the nerves surrounding the hippocampus become tangled , nerve impulses no longer carry information to or from the brain. The brain's circuits are now disconnected and information cannot be retrieved. This entanglement does not destroy the memory stored information, it prevents the information from being transferred. See acetylcarnitine and indomethacin in this section.

REFERENCES

Acarosan, 1994, by Center Laboratories, Port Washington, NY.

Aging, Long Life & Better Health, 1994, by Dr. W. Lamar Rosquist, N.D.,D.C.

A Guide To Understanding Psoriasis, 1995, by National Psoriasis Foundation.

ALOE VERA A Mission Discovered, 1993, by Lee Ritter.

Alternative Medicine The Definitive Guide, 1994, by Deepak Chopra, M.D. Compiled by The Burton Goldberg Group.

Alternative Medicine Yellow Pages, 1995, by Future Medicine Publishing, Inc.

Alzheimer's Disease, 1994, National Institute of Mental Health

Antioxidant, The, 1993, by Gail L. Becker, R.D.

Anxiety Disorders, September 1994, National Institutes of Health, National Institute of Mental Health.

Apple Cider Vinegar (Voted #1 Home Remedy by "Your Health Readers"). By Edward Ward, 1994. Globe Communications Corp.,5401 NW Broken Sound Blvd., Boca, Raton, FL 33487.

Apple Cider Vinegar Health System, by Paul C. Bragg, N.D., Ph.D & Patricia Bragg, N.D., Ph.D

A Remarkable Medicine Has Been Overlooked, 1981, by Dreyfus Medical Foundation.

Are Your Dental Fillings Poisoning You?, 1986, by Guy S. Fasciana, D. M.D.

Army Echoes, July-September 1995, Jan-March 1996, Army Retirement Services.

Atlanta Journal\Constitution, The, 21 November 1994.

A Wellness Way of Life, 1991, 2nd Edition. Robbins, Power, & Burgess, WCB Brown & Benchmark.

Beano Bulletin, Vol. 3, No. 4, Fall 1995.

Before You Call the Doctor, 1992, by Anne Simmons, M.D., Bobbie Hasselbring and Michael Castleman.

Belleville Journal, page 5A, 22 March 1995. "Back Talk" by Dr. Warren A. Stewart, Jr.

Blacks Medical Dictionary, 35th Edition, 1987, edited by C.W.H. Harvard.

Bottom Line Year Book 1995 & 1996, by the Editors of Bottom Line, Boardroom Classics.

Brain, The, 1984, by Richard Restak, M.D.

Cancer Facts for Men, 1990, 90-1.5MM-Rev.4/93-No.2007, Amercan Cancer Society, Inc.

Cancer Facts for Women, 1990, 90-1.5MM-Rev. 10/94-No.2008, American Cancer Society, Inc.

Cancer of the Lung Research Report, February 1993, National Cancer Institute.

Carpal Tunnel Syndrome, *Prevention & Treatment*, 1994, by Kate Montgomery.

Chelation Therapy, 1984, by Dr. Morton Walker.

Choices - Realistic Alternatives in Cancer Treatment, 1987, by Marion Morra & Eve Potts.

Cholesterol - A Guide to Low-Cholesterol Living 1990. Krames Communications, San Bruno, CA.

City Utilities of Springfield, MO, 1994, 417-863-9000. Carbon Monoxide Brochure.

COLLOIDAL SILVER The Amazing Alternative to Antibiotics, 1994, by The Association for Advanced Colloid Research.

Complete Guide to Mercury Toxicity from Dental Fillings, The, 1988, by Joyal Taylor D.D.S.

Complete & Up-to-Date FAT Book, The, 1993, by Karen J. Bellerson.

Complex Carbohydrate Handbook, The 1981, by Shirley Ross.

Consumer Reports, July 1995, A Publication of Consumers Union.

Cures from the Last Chance Clinic, 1995, published by The University of Natural Healing, Inc.

Cut Your Cholesterol 30 Points in 30 Days (a drug-free doctor-approved plan) 1994. James O'Brien, Globe Communications Corp., 5401 NW Broken sound Blvd., Boca Raton, FL 33487.

DETOX, 1984, by Phyllis Saifer, M.D., M.P.H., and Merla Zellerbach.

Dial An Expert, 1986, by Susan Osborn.

Diet, Nutrition & Cancer Prevention: The Good News 1987, U.S. Department of Health and Human Services.

Dietary Guidelines for Americans, Third Edition, November 1990. Home and Garden Bulletin # 232, U.S. Department of Agriculture, U.S. Department of Health and Human Services.

Disease Free, 1993, by Matthew Hoffman, William Le Gro and the editors of Prevention Magazine Health Books.

Doctor's Book of Home Remedies, The, 1993, by Sid Kirchheimer and the editors of Prevention Magazine Health Books.

Dorland's Illustrated Medical Dictionary, 27th Edition, 1985. W.B. Saunders Company, Harcourt Brace Jovanovich, Inc.

Dr. Atkins' New Diet Revolution, 1992, by Robert C. Atkins.

Eating Disorders, January 1993, U.S. Department of health and Human Services, National Institute of Mental Health.

Eight-Week Cholesterol Cure, The, 1989, by Robert E. Kowalski.

Encyclopedia of Health, The - Nutrition, 1991, by Dale C. Garell, M.D.

Encyclopedia of Organic Gardening, 1978, by the staff of Organic Gardening magazine.

Facing Forward, A Guide for Cancer Survivors, October 1992, National Cancer Institute, U.S. Department of Health and Human Services.

Family Circle, February 1, 1995, Can Vitamins Save Your Life? (pages 28 & 29).

Family Guide To Natural Medicine, 1993, Reader's Digest Association Inc.

Family Medical Guide & Health Handbook, 1995, by the Editors of Consumer Guide.

Fat Burning Foods, 1995, compiled by K. Patricia Stone, M.S., R.D.

Food - Cooking Advice is Just a Phone Call Away, November 8, 1995, St Louis Post Dispatch.

Food Pharmacy, The, 1988, by Jean Carper.

Foods That Make You Lose Weight or Negative Calories, 1990, by Isabelle Martin.

Garlic, The Miracle Herb, 1995, by Judy Lin Eftekhar, Globe Communications Corp., 5401 NW Broken sound Blvd., Boca Raton, FL 33487.

Guide to a Healthier Diet, The--*Eat Well/Be Well*, 1988. Dr. Elaine Fox, Distron Video Corporation, P.O. Box 1040, New Hyde Park, N.Y. 11040.

Healing, Foods, The, 1989, by Patricia Hausman & Judith Benn Hurley.

Healing Powers of Chelation Therapy, The, 1985, by John Parks Trowbridge, M.D. & Morton Walker, D.P.M.

Health Alternatives, 1991, by Alex Duarte, O.D,, Ph.D.

Health Food Dictionary and Recipes, The, by Anstice Carroll and Embree De Persiis Vona.

Health & Healing, Tomorrow's Medicine Today, by Dr. Julian Whitaker, Phillips Publishing, Inc., 7811 Montrose Road, Suite 200, Potomac, Maryland 20854.

Help Yourself to Good Health. Presented in the public interest by the National Institute on Aging and by Pfizer Pharmaceuticals.

Herbally Yours, 1982, by Penny C. Royal.

Here's to Your Health Newsletter, Vol. 5, No. 7, July 1995, Heart Foods Company Inc.

Home Remedies Handbook, The, by the Editors of Consumer Guide with John E. Renner, M.D., and the Consumer Health Information Research Institute.

Household Environment and Chronic Illness, The, 1980, edited by Guy O. Pfeiffer, M.D., Casimir M. Nikel, F.A.C.H.A., with forward by Richard Mackarness, M.B., B.S., D.P.M.

How to Be Your Own Nutritionist, 1987, by Stuart M. Berger, M.D.

How to Reverse Aging, 1995, by James O'Brien, Globe Communications Corp., 5401 NW Broken sound Blvd., Boca Raton, FL 33487.

How to Stay Out of The Doctor's Office, 1992, Dr. Edward M. Wagner with Sylvia Goldfarb.

INFOCUS, Volume 3, Number 4, pages 1 & 8, American Autoimmune Related Diseases Association, Inc.

"I See It... But I Still Don't Believe It!" The Amazing Story of Catalyst Water 1987.

It's All in Your Head - Diseases Caused by Silver-Mercury Fillings, 1990, by Hal A. Huggins, DDS.

Is "Modern" Medicine Killing You, 1995, by Dr. Marcus Laux, (Naturally Well-).

Journal of Longevity Research, Volume 1/No. 10, 1995.

Ladies Home Journal, August 1995, page 47.

Matthew Lesko Info Power I & II and brochures, 1994.

McCalls Magazine, May 1995, Page 56; August 1992, page 42 & 52.

Medical Advances, 1977, by Lawrence Galton.

Medical Dictionary, 1987, Websters New World, Stedman's.

Mercury Contamination: A Human Tragedy, 1977, by Patricia A. D'Itri and Frank M. D'Itri.

Miracle of Garlic and Vinegar, The, 1993 & 1995. James O'Brien, Globe Communications Corporation, 5401 N.W. Broken Sound Blvd., Boca Raton, FL 33487.

Modern Maturity, March-April 1995, pages 18 and 62 to 66.

Myotherapy - Bonnie Prudden's Complete Guide to Pain-Free Living, 1984, by Bonnie Prudden.

National Wildlife Federation brochure, December 1995.

Natural Way, The. July 1995.

Nature's Healing Herbs, 1994, James O'Brien, Globe Communications Corporation, 5401 N.W. Broken Sound Blvd., Boca Raton, FL 33487

Ninety Days to Self-Healing, 1977, by C. Norman Shealy, M.D.

Nontoxic & Natural, 1984, by Debra Lynn Dadd.

Ozarks Senior Living, Volume 4, No. 12, January 1995.

Pork, A Key to Good Health, Illinois Pork Producers Association & American Heart Association of Metropolitan Chicago & Illinois Affiliate.

Prescription for Nutritional Healing, 1990, by James F. Balch, M.D. & Phyllis A. Balch, C.N.C.

Prevention's Guide to Health, For Men Only, page 32, December 1995, Rodale Press, Inc.

Product and Service Guide, 1995, Terrace International Distributors, Inc.

Rainforest, 1991, by Lois Warburton

Reader's Digest Illustrated Encyclopedia Dictionary A thru Z, 1987, The Reader's Digest Association, Inc., Pleasantville, New York.

Remedy, November\December 1994, pages 18-31.

Reverse the Aging Process Naturally, 1993, Gary Null and Martin Feldman, M.D.

Reversing Heart Disease, 1990, by Dean Ornish, M.D.

Roger's Recovery from AIDS, 1993, by Bob Owen Ph.D.

Running & FitNews, November 1994.

Shiatsu, 1974, by Tokujiro Namikoshi.

Sixty Percent of Deaths from Cancer May Be Preventable, 1993, 93-10MM-No. 7099, American Cancer Society, Inc.

Spirulina, The Whole Food Revolution, 1982, by Larry Switzer.

Substance Abuse and Its Prevention, 1992, by Mary Lou Jones, ACSW and Patrick Jones, CAC, ACSW.

SuperLearning, 1979, by Sheila Ostrander and Lynn Schroeder with Nancy Ostrander.

SuperMemory, 1991, by Sheila Ostrander and Lynn Schroeder with Nancy Ostrander.

Supernutrition for Healthy Hearts, 1975, by Richard Passwater, Ph.D.

Taber's Cyclopedia Medical Dictionary, 1989, F.A. Davis Company.

Think Yourself Well, 1995, by Bernard Ward, Globe Digest.

Ultimate Diet Tool Kit, The, 1994, by Stanford Apseloff & Glen Apseloff, M.D.

United States Army Health Services Command. Brochure 1991.

U.S. News & World Report, June 20, 1994, pages 66-68; March 27, 1995, pages 48-58.

More Survival Kindle E-Books And Survival Paperback Books For YOU!

Joseph A. Laydon Jr. (MSG Ret. Army) is the author and owner of Intensive Research Information Services And Products (IRISAP). Joseph has been writing "self-reliance" orientated data since 1991 and since July 2012 has been re-publishing his works via Kindle E-Books and CreateSpace Paperback Books. He has self-published more than **80+ Survival Books** (Kindle E-Books and Paperback Books). Below is a list of all his Survival Books and you can see these books by simply going to the 02 websites listed below for detailed descriptions and videos. See *"About Author."*

- **Kindle E-Books:**--------------------**www.survivalexpertebooks.com**

- **Paperback Books:**-----------------**www.survivalexpertbooks.com**

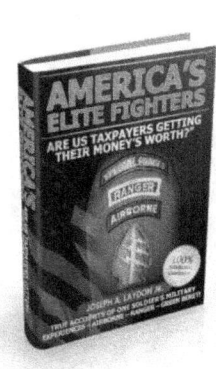 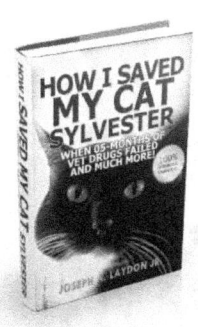 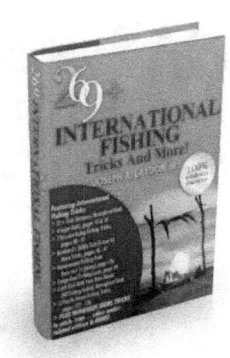

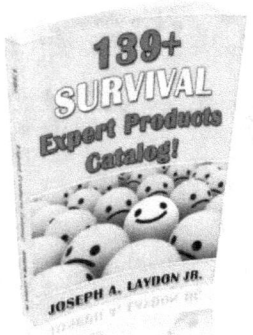

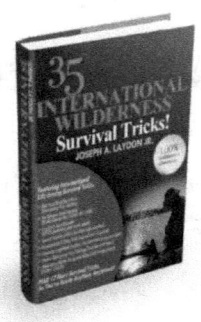

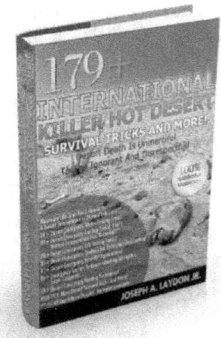

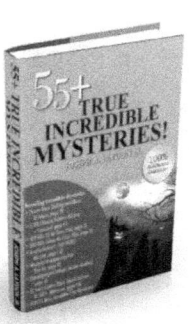

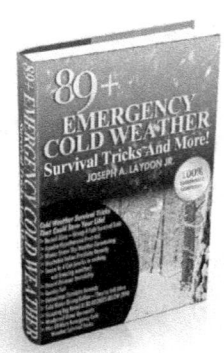

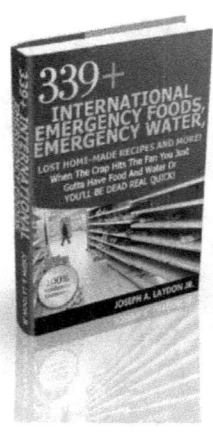

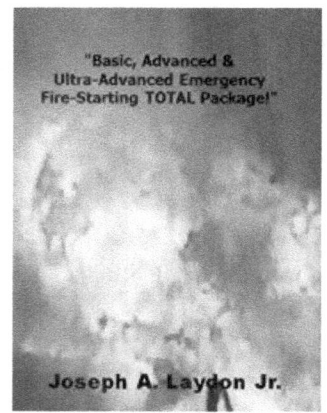

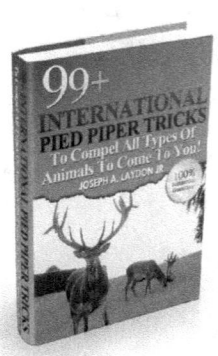

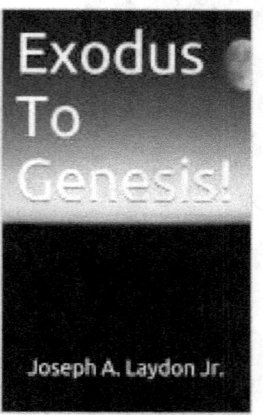

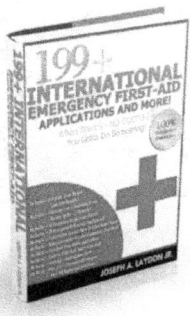

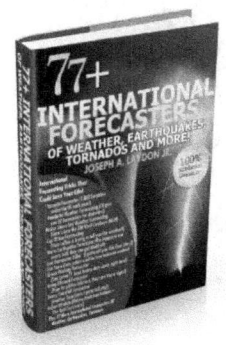

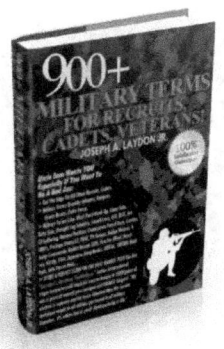

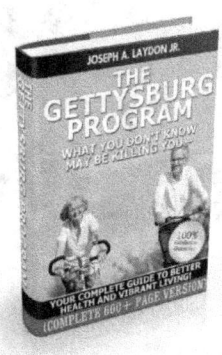

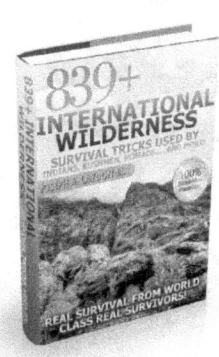

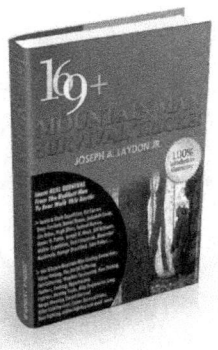

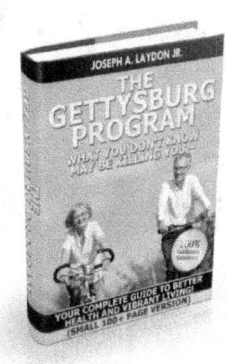

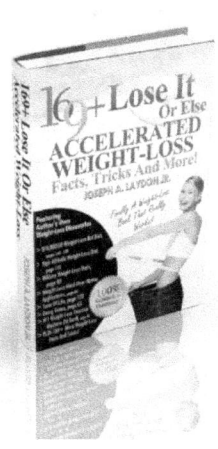

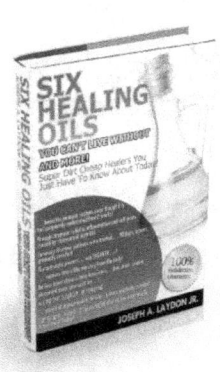

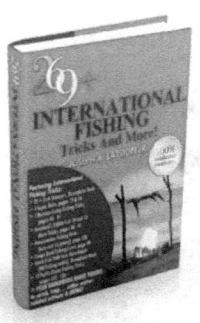

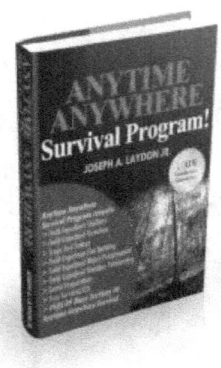

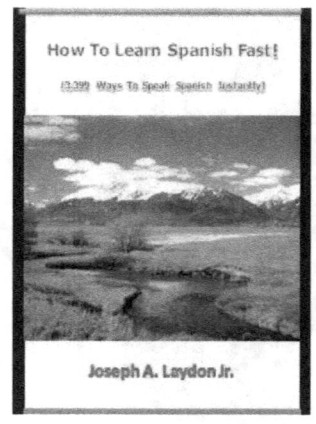

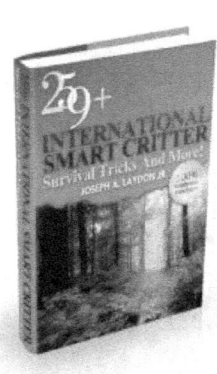

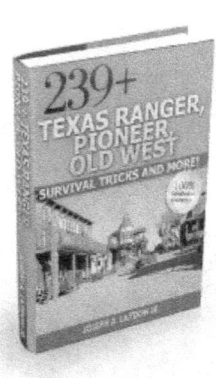

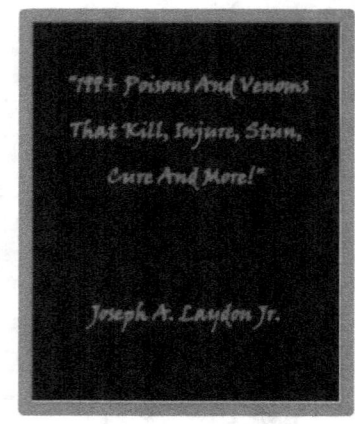

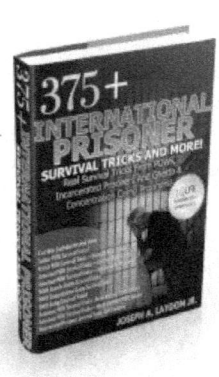

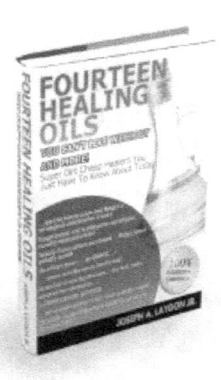

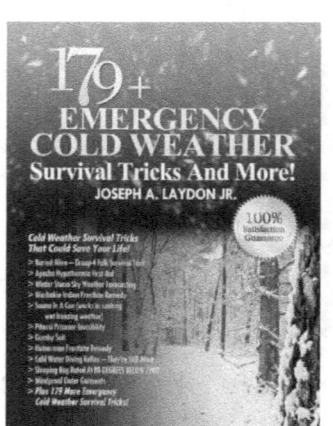

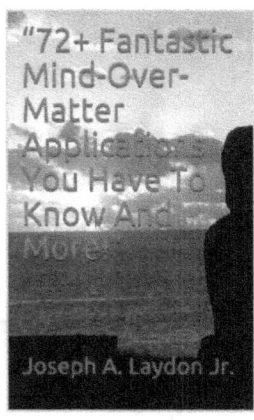

"72+ Fantastic Mind-Over-Matter Applications You Have To Know And More!

Joseph A. Laydon Jr.

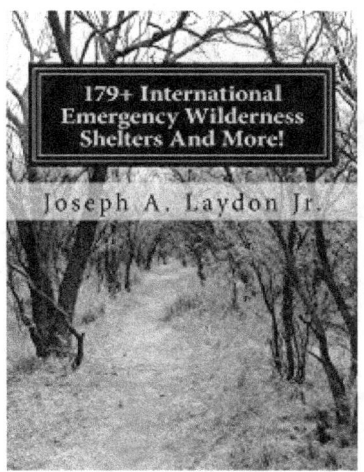

179+ International Emergency Wilderness Shelters And More!

Joseph A. Laydon Jr.

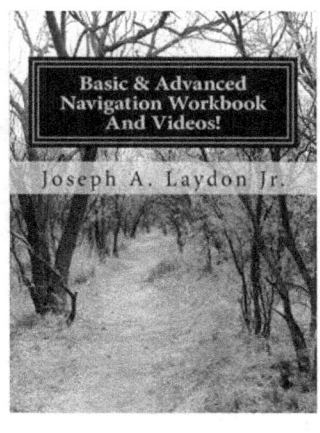

Basic & Advanced Navigation Workbook And Videos!

Joseph A. Laydon Jr.

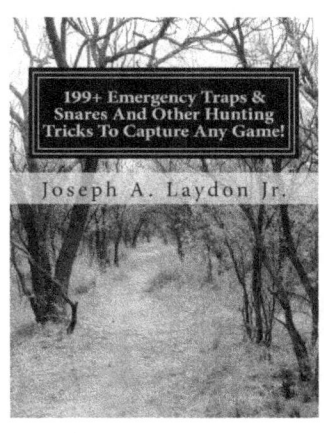

199+ Emergency Traps & Snares And Other Hunting Tricks To Capture Any Game!

Joseph A. Laydon Jr.

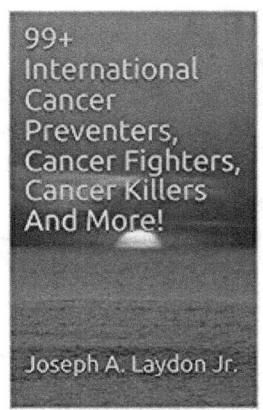

99+ International Cancer Preventers, Cancer Fighters, Cancer Killers And More!

Joseph A. Laydon Jr.

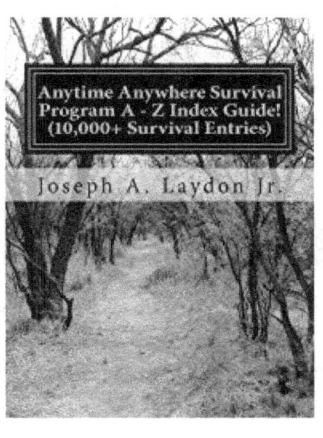

Anytime Anywhere Survival Program A - Z Index Guide! (10,000+ Survival Entries)

Joseph A. Laydon Jr.

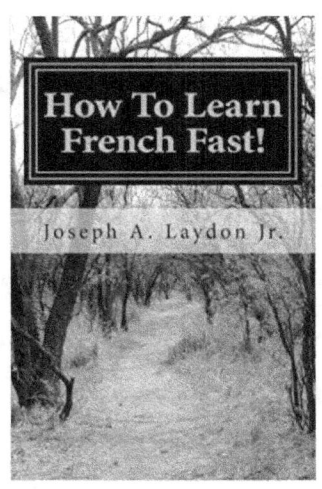

How To Learn French Fast!

Joseph A. Laydon Jr.

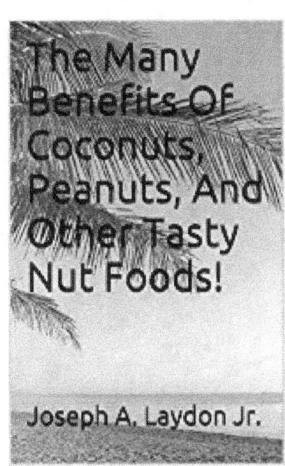

The Many Benefits Of Coconuts, Peanuts, And Other Tasty Nut Foods!

Joseph A. Laydon Jr.

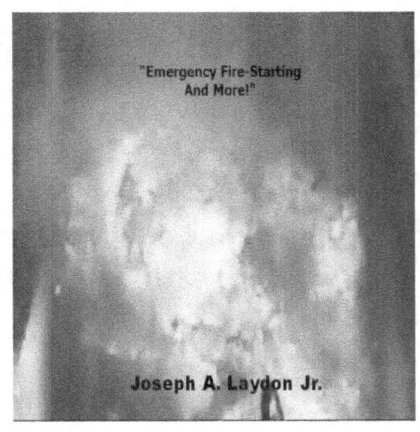

"Emergency Fire-Starting And More!"

Joseph A. Laydon Jr.

About The Author

Joseph A. Laydon Jr. (MSG Ret. Army – 18Z5V) is the author and owner of
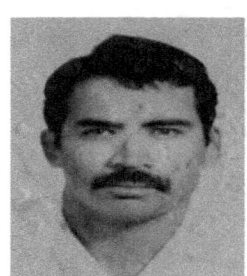
Intensive Research Information Services And Products (IRISAP). Joseph is a well-qualified instructor in international wilderness survival and the other 03 Survivals he teaches (Health, Crime, and Money). He is a 20-year US Army veteran (Master Sergeant E-8 - 18Z5V) associated with all Special Operations units in the US military, as well as Special Ops units in the Mid-East and Central & South America.

He's a qualified SERE Instructor (Survival Evasion Resistance & Escape) and has **taught wilderness survival** at the college level for 03 years. He's a qualified instructor in basic & advanced pistol marksmanship, basic & advanced rifle marksmanship, CQB (Close Quarter Battle), basic & advanced cross-country navigation, basic mountaineering techniques, and self-defense. Since 1994, he's published many self-improvement Survival Programs, Survival Videos, SPECIAL Reports, Intelligence Reports, monthly Newsletters, **80+ Survival Books** (Kindle E-Books & CreateSpace Paperback Books) and more in the works.

He's an inventor, he *"sideways engineers"* new survival tricks that can SAVE YOUR LIFE! An example: On 17 August 2000 - 1417 hours, at Scott Lake, Scott AFB, IL, Joseph made international history! He is the 1st in the world to replicate the mysterious fires of Africa using a single drop of water! On 05 January 2001, he discovered how to start a life-saving fire in just 02-seconds using a beam of light from a flashlight in pitch black *"blind man"* darkness! On 06 April 2005 - 1810 hours, he invented delicious & tasty Solid Fuel Rolls and several Trail-Mix Cookies that are used as emergency foods and used as long-burning emergency fire-starting kindling.

And recently - **50+ MORE TOP SECRET INVENTIONS** of advanced & ultra-advanced fire-starting like starting EMERGENCY FIRE-STARTING using personal care products and first-aid products you already use like:

- Shampoo
- Toothpastes
- Mouthwashes
- Breath Drops & Breath Sprays
- Salves
- Ointments
- Over-The-Counter Medicines
- Drink Enhancement Products
- Other ingredients like your spit (saliva), your urination,...

See **www.survivalexpert.com/fire**

He also teaches Advanced Navigation (*Basic & Advanced Navigation Workbook And Videos* [includes Workbook, Videos, maps, protractors,…]) so you're ready Anytime Anywhere! Only from IRISAP and only for privileged IRISAP subscribers - YOU! See *Basic & Advanced Navigation Workbook And Videos* at

www.survivalexpertbooks.com/navigation

Below is a sample of his military achievements & qualifications (**not in chronological order**) which reflect his unique & superior ability to teach basic, advanced & ultra-advanced survival applications, techniques and "tricks" that could help you AVOID serious killer survival threats as well as SAVE YOUR LIFE when you get in life or death situations. His trade secrets, Programs, and Videos are only offered to IRISAP subscribers-YOU!

- US Army Airborne School
- US Army Special Forces Qualification Course - SFQC (Green Beret)
- US Army Master Parachutist Wings
- Uruguayan Parachutist Wings
- British Parachutist Wings
- Kingdom of Jordan Parachutist Wings
- Expert Infantry Badge - EIB
- 82nd Airborne Division Recondo Course
- Adverse Weather Aerial Delivery System Tests - AWADS (01 of 386 volunteer paratroopers)
- US Army Special Forces Weapons Course (US & foreign pistols, submachineguns, assault rifles, rifles, machineguns, mortars, anti-tank weapons, anti-aircraft weapons,…)
- Weapons Armorer Course
- Indirect Fire Course (60mm, 81mm, & 4.2 inch *"four deuce"* mortars)
- Jumpmaster Course
- Basic French Language Course
- Combat Infantry Badge - CIB
- US Army Ranger Course
- Advanced Navigation Course
- Special Forces Sniper Course (02)
- Survival Evasion Resistance and Escape Instructor Course (SERE Level B)
- Wilderness Survival Instructor (College level - 03 years / 1991 - 1994)
- Rappell Master
- Fast Rope Master
- International Sniper Instructor
- International Close Quarter Battle (CQB) Instructor
- Participated In Multiple Combat Actions

- Special Forces Operations And Intelligence Course (O&I)
- Good Conduct Medal (06)
- Army Commendation Medal
- Army Achievement Medal (02)
- Meritorious Service Medal (02)
- Armed Forces Expeditionary Medal
- Letters Of Commendation (13)
- Letters Of Appreciation (08)
- Held **SECRET and TOP SECRET Clearances** for 20+ years

Featured on FOX-2 (24 August 2000). Joseph now resides in Illinois. He offers products concerning Wilderness Survival, Health Survival, Crime Survival, and Money Survival so to greatly enhance the lives of all IRISAP subscribers - YOU! Any questions, write to Joseph today.

Sincerely,
Joseph A. Laydon Jr. (IRISAP)
P.O. Box 48
Cutler, IL 62238-0048

You And Yours Have A Safe One
Anytime Anywhere,

Joseph A. Laydon Jr.

E-Mail: wwwsurvivalexpert@yahoo.com

WEBSITES

- Main Website----------------------------www.survivalexpert.com
- 40+ Survival Paperback Books-----------www.survivalexpertbooks.com
- 40+ Survival Kindle E-Books------------www.survivalexpertebooks.com
- Anytime Anywhere Survival--------------www.anytimeanywheresurvival.com
- Weight-Loss----------------------------www.loseitorelseweightloss.com
- True Scary Videos (all FREE)-----------www.truescaryvideos.com
- Exodus To Genesis----------------------www.exodustogenesis.com

Take Notes

Take Notes

Take Notes

Take Notes

Take Notes

Take Notes

Take Notes

Take Notes

"Survival Expert Private Mailing List!"

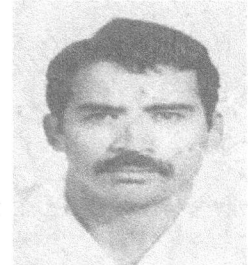

THANK YOU for your wise interest in this Survival Book. I have 80+ more Survival Books (Paperback Books & Kindle E-Books) that I've written and can be found at www.amazon.com See **www.survivalexpertbooks.com** and **www.survivalexpertebooks.com** for descriptions and videos on my books. And yes, I wrote every single word of each Survival Book. See *About The Author*.

Now let's get to my mailing list. How would you like get on my private 'Survival Expert' mailing list? NO, this isn't an e-mail list offer. This is a real – in your hands mailing list via the good ol' United States Postal Service.

I will cover the following subjects for each monthly mail-out:

- **Wilderness Survival:** I have THOUSANDS and THOUSANDS of real international survival tricks from the REAL SURVIVORS throughout the world and throughout history. Forget that worthless - 'will get you killed' - survival crap on television.

- **Health Survival:** I started my Health Survival back in the late 1990s. I study the stuff like I'm going to college. But I focus on dozens and dozens of Alternative Therapies. Here, let me tell you something that happened to me a couple years ago. A doctor in Sparta, IL told me 04-times, 04-times – quote: *"You have three weeks to live."* Hey, I'm still here. I'll tell you all about it PLUS a ton more of REAL Health Survival that's worthy of your attention for a healthy vibrant life.

- **Crime Survival:** Hey, you can be a bad ass in the woods and healthy as a horse but what about all those pieces of sh!+ cowards out there that will steal your money, hurt you, kill you or hurt & kill your loved ones in your home. I'll give you the Facts Of Life when it comes to Crime Survival and how to AVOID it and / or remedy it.

- **Money Survival:** We can all use more cash but I gotta tell you, most (95%) of that 'Make Money From Home' – excuse my language, is pure Bull Shit. They're all scams run by scumbags. And the few that are legit, it's still worthless. Why? Cause they can't teach. They just confuse and frustrate you till you give up. Now here's where I come in. I make some money via the internet. But most of my stuff on the internet are like Business Cards. People go to my several websites to check out that I'm a real person and they can see that I really do have my own Survival Products.

If you're interested in starting / re-starting your own home-based business and learning some super simple & unique applications that I use all the time and you're interested in the other Survivals - Wilderness Survival, Health Survival and Crime Survival, read my FREE OFFER. On the next few pages is my **FREE OFFER** for YOU. **DON'T SEND ME ANY MONEY**. Check out my **FREE OFFER** below.

"DO NOT SEND ME ANY MONEY. I Will Send You Any 03 Of 10 Survival Tricks Of Your Choice At NO-CHARGE!"

WILDERNESS-SURVIVAL   HEALTH-SURVIVAL   CRIME-SURVIVAL   MONEY-SURVIVAL

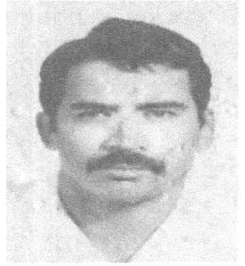

Hello, my name is Joseph A. Laydon Jr. (Cutler, IL). Since 1991 I've been teaching good folks like you REAL international survival. I have very satisfied customers from Canada to South Africa.

I will send you **any 03 international survival tricks of your choice** that you can use to AVOID trouble in the first place and get you out of trouble when your life and the lives of your loved ones are on the line.

Here's a quick list of all 10 Survival Tricks so You're Ready Anytime Anywhere. Somebody has to be the hero, why not YOU! OK, here's the list:

- PRSC
- Sauna In A Can!
- Home Invasion Defense!
- Laydon's Burn Remedy!
- Snakebite & Brown Recluse Spider Bite Remedy!
- Starting An Emergency Fire - Rub Your Shoe On A Rock!
- Panamanian Fishing Trick (100 Fish)!
- 100% Accurate Weather Forecasting Trick!
- Goose Final Approach!
- No Weapon Duck Hunting!

Private Message & Bonus
**www.survivalexpertbooks.com/
private-list**
(Special Bonus Just For YOU)

Now here are the descriptions for each of the 10 survival tricks. I will send you any 03 survival tricks of your choice - FREE - AT NO CHARGE!

Why? Cause once you see the great quality of the survival tricks you pick, I know you'll want all the others listed here PLUS 100 more for the small cost of a double cheeseburger, large fries and large coke. I'll send you 100+ more survival tricks so You're Ready Anytime Anywhere! OK, let's get started with the 10 international survival tricks. I'll send you any 03 of your choice FREE At NO-CHARGE! Let's start with *PRSC*.

01) PRSC!: I've had customers thank me for sending them *PRSC*. One customer wrote me and asked if I knew **how many lives I've saved with PRSC.**

PRSC is an acronym used by US Army Infantry units during their planning for combat missions. *PRSC* is used to keep soldiers from getting killed. I 'civilianized' *PRSC* for you and I have been teaching *PRSC* since the mid-1990s. *PRSC* could SAVE YOUR LIFE and the lives under your care.

I hear about outdoor tragedies (deaths) happening all the time and I nod my head thinking '*if they used PRSC*' or was one of my subscribers, **they'd be alive today.**' I'll tell you all about *PRSC* once you give me your go ahead to send you **any 03 survival tricks of your choice!**

02) Sauna In A Can!: I entered the US Army and was in the Infantry assigned to the 82nd Airborne out of Fort Bragg, NC. I gotta tell you, Airborne Infantry is a miserable miserable job and on top of that we jumped out of C-130 aircraft at 1 o'clock in the morning loaded down with all kinds of gear, severely nauseated and we were always cold and soaking wet. Back then, there was no fancy Goretex to keep us dry.

Well during a 03-week Recondo School I was attending, I was assigned Assistant Patrol Leader. We were out in the woods in the dead of winter learning patrolling. That North Carolina cold is a wet cold, a humid cold and it goes right thru you - it stings, it hurts. Anyway, I was going around the perimeter making sure the patrol members weren't sleeping. Everybody was cold and miserable in our foxholes. But one Private kept smiling up at me every time I passed by his foxhole.

Finally I whispered something like 'what is wrong with you?

Why aren't you miserable like the rest of us?' He then told me he was toasty warm and what he was doing and after I graduated from that course, I started using it too and used it throughout my military career. I nicknamed it *Sauna In A Can*. And it works even if you're shivering soaking wet and you're freezing to death! How does it work? I'll tell you EVERYTHING once I get your OK to send you **any 03 survival tricks!**

03) Home Invasion Defense!: Between 2003 and 2007, an estimated 3,700,000 homes were burglarized on average in the US. And about 28% of the time, home owners were present during the burglary. The term home invasion has been broadened to other home crimes besides simple burglary. **Before I carry-on, read that folded-up page attached to this letter.**

You'll see that I was an international sniper instructor and an international Close Quarter Battle (CQB) instructor. I took part in many many high risk and challenging training exercises and combat missions. I always thought the training was far more dangerous than the combat missions I participated in.

I learned a great deal and I will share some of it with you. I want to show you how to defend yourself in your own home when an uninvited invader(s) enters your home to do you and your loved ones some serious harm. You have the right to defend yourself.

And you MUST DEFEND yourself & your loved ones or everyone will end up to be another set of DEAD STATISTICS.

⬇
Private Message & Bonus
www.survivalexpertbooks.com/
private-list
(Special Bonus Just For YOU)
⬆

I'll show you some simple tactics that really work that are used by America's military elite units like:
- US Army Delta Force
- US Navy SEALs
- Special A-Teams (Green Berets)
- US Army Rangers
- Special Teams of the US Marine Corps

How can you take-on 01 or more intruders in your home? I'll tell you everything when I send you 03 of these survival tricks FREE!

04) Laydon's Super Quick Burn & Pain Remedy!: Everybody has their own home remedies for this or that. But I will tell you 1st hand:
On 01 Oct. 2006, I stopped the **POUNDING PAIN** after I spilled boiling hot tea directly on my left hand & wrist.

This **super cheap** ingredient worked so good, the **POUNDING PAIN STOPPED** in just 120 seconds flat and never returned and weeks later there were no scars.

It could only happen to me. On 04 Sep. 2015, I was cleaning up my carport. What I didn't know was there was a wasp nest inside a large hose I had hanging up. I reached underneath it and got stung on all 05 fingers of my left hand.

The **PAIN WAS SO AGONIZING** I thought I hit a live wire but there were no live wires.

Like a sissy boy I sprinted to my house and glancing behind me were a few wasps in trail. I went to my medicine cabinet and applied this same cheap ingredient and **IT STOPPED THE POUNDING PAIN IN ALL MY FIVE FINGERS!**

Getting stung 05-times at the same time by multiple wasps would send most people to the hospital. With a co-pay, you're probably out a $100 bucks easy. Not me, I used this super cheap ingredient for just a few bucks. I'm telling you, this super cheap ingredient works so good for STOPPING POUNDING PAIN super quick for:
- Severe burns
- Wasps stings
- Cuts

This super cheap ingredient WORKS SO GOOD it should be in every medicine cabinet, every ambulance, every fire truck, every emergency room, **in your medicine cabinet**,… but it's not.

I have at least 02 of these in my medicine cabinet standing by at all times. And I'll tell you everything once I get your OK to send you your choice of survival tricks!

05) Snakebite & Brown Recluse Spider Bite Remedy!: You don't have to be out in the wilderness to be tagged by venomous snakes. And those venomous Brown Recluse spiders, Black Widow spiders,…are everywhere.

Good folks all over the world purchase my Survival Programs. Many times I talk to folks that are already survival experts in their own right and I am challenged to send them a quality Survival Product.

One day I was talking on the phone to one of my subscribers. Like me, he worked in the jungles of Central America. Initially I thought he was B.S.ing me till he proved himself by saying key things.

Anyway he told me a story of how he learned about a venomous snakebite remedy that is **so effective** it even works **INSTANTLY** for venomous spiders like the Brown Recluse, Black Widow,…

What if you or your loved ones got tagged by a venomous snake or got tagged by a venomous spider and there are NO IMMEDIATE EMERGENCY SERVICES available? You'll know what to do you send me your choice of Survival Tricks.

06) Starting An Emergency Fire – Rub Your Shoe On A Rock!:

I can tell you many true stories where regular folks got in trouble outdoors and froze to death. Some were found with matches on them yet they couldn't start a fire to literally save their lives. I consider myself an expert in emergency fire-starting. Why?

First of all **I DO NOT TEACH** any of the 'rubbing 02 sticks together' field-craft. Why? Too dang hard to get to work. 2nd, that 'rubbing 02 sticks together' will NEVER NEVER NEVER NEVER WORK if you're truly hypothermic. Trust me.

Private Message & Bonus
www.survivalexpertbooks.com/
private-list
(Special Bonus Just For YOU)

There's nothing wrong with taking matches and lighters out in the woods with you. But folks have been found DEAD DEAD with matches and lighters on them, yet they couldn't start a fire to literally save their life. I have INVENTED many basic, advanced and ultra-advanced emergency fire-starting applications than you could use on several dozen camping trips.

And one of my many many emergency fire-starting inventions is *Rub Your Shoe On A Rock*. This really works and if you're so hypothermic your hands and fingers will not work. You can't even pull up your zipper or button your coat – your hands and fingers will not work. So using matches and lighters is impossible. And forget about 'rubbing 02 sticks together.' No bloody way. Using *Rub Your Shoe On A Rock*, you're using the weight of your body to start an emergency fire.

Of all the *8 Elements of Survival* (Fire, Water, Shelter, First-Aid, Signal, Food, Weapons and Navigation) – in my humble opinion, FIRE is the most important in most survival situations. And this unknown fire-starting trick could save your life and those under your care! How does it work? I'll give you all the life-saving details when I send you your choice of Survival Tricks.

07) Panamanian Fishing Trick (100 Fish)!:

Do you like eating breaded fish filets? MMmmmmmm! I surely do. This is not a 'fish story.' This is a true story. For about 05-years, back in the 1980s and early 1990s I was stationed at Fort Davis, Panama with a battalion of Army Special Forces (Green Berets) soldiers.

On very rare occasions when the entire battalion was together, we'd have a fish fry. We're talking about 18 A-Teams plus Headquarters company (200+), that's a lot of hungry soldiers.

Where in the heck are they going to get all the fish to feed all these hungry soldiers? I didn't care where the fish came from, I was hungry. Man those breaded fish filets were very very tasty.

Well the years I was down there, I kept hearing the same story of these 02 soldiers from Headquarters Company going out on a boat to Gatun Lake (supports the Panama Canal) and between 7am and about 12 noon, those 02 soldiers would **ALWAYS ALWAYS CATCH ABOUT 100 BASS FISH – GUARANTEED!**

'No way' I thought, it's B.S.

Well towards the end of my tour (July 1991), I decided to track down those 02 soldiers and find out how they were catching 100 bass fish in just 04 hours or so.

Well I tracked them down and they told me exactly what they were LEGALLY doing to catch 100 bass fish (no fish limit in Panama).

Days later I tried it myself just off the bank on Gatun Lake and **BAMM!**

In just a couple minutes, I got me a tasty bass fish real quick. I named this fishing trick - the *Panamanian Fishing Trick*. <u>How does it work?</u> And I'll tell you everything once I get your OK to send you your choice of FREE Survival Tricks.

08) 100% Accurate Weather Forecasting Trick!: Here's a stone cold fact - Mother Nature and all She possesses is the MOST POWERFUL FORCE on Earth. More powerful than all the nukes ever built. And one of the wraths of Mother Nature is weather. I'm going to send you a weather forecasting trick that is 100% accurate! You gotta know when a storm is heading your way. Storms of all sorts hurt & kill people all across the globe <u>EVERY MINUTE OF THE DAY</u>!!! You can use this weather forecasting trick in the woods or even in the city in just 02-seconds. <u>How does it work?</u> I'll tell you everything with your permission to send you any 03 survival tricks.

09) Goose Final Approach!: I use to work at a US government site that required me to have a **TOP SECRET** Security Clearance. It took me a year and a half to get it but I got it. One day while working there, I was talking to one of the janitors. We were talking about hunting and he told me his friend would catch geese without any hunting at all. The geese would fly to him and he'd put that critter on

the dinner table. He didn't believe him so his friend invited him out to his house out in the country. Not long after he arrived at his friend's house - **BAMM!** Another goose for the dinner table. When he told me this story, I was amazed but thought - *'talk about thinking outside the box.'* I named this 'no hunting trick' - *Goose Final Approach*.

Private Message & Bonus
www.survivalexpertbooks.com/
private-list
(Special Bonus Just For YOU)

Even World Class hunters don't know about this ingenious 'no hunting trick.' I asked him what about ducks. It's works on ducks too? He didn't know. So here's *'No Weapon Duck Hunting.'*

10) No Weapon Duck Hunting!: I don't know if you've ever tasted duck - it's DELICIOUS! Tastier than chicken, tuna, angus beef, all beef hot dogs,… Here's a real neat survival trick to catch all the ducks you can eat. And I'll explain why it works. I call it *'No Weapon Duck Hunting.'* You:
- Don't need a shotgun
- Don't need a Bola
- Don't need a Duck Call
- Don't need a Trap
- Don't need a Blind

I'll tell you everything once you give me your permission to send you your choice of international survival tricks at absolutely NO-CHARGE.

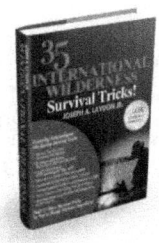
The title of this book is *"35 International Wilderness Survival Tricks!"* - but there are actually 100+ Survival Tricks included in this Survival Book!

I don't advertise the actual number of survival tricks. Only to YOU, a potential customer. And when **YOU PICK YOUR CHOICE OF ANY 03 SURVIVAL TRICKS**, you'll get a good taste of all 100+ survival tricks in this Survival Book. And it's just 01 of my **80+ Survival Books** (Paperback Books & Kindle E-Books - I'm the original writer - no ghost writers).

Included is a website page. It tells you that I'm a real person and I'll send you your choice of survival tricks - FREE at NO CHARGE! PLUS, <u>I HAVE A BONUS WAITING FOR YOU!</u> So go ahead and:
- Go to the website page listed above
- See *'About The Author'*
- Send in Order Form today (next two pages after Testimonials)

Here are couple Testimonials before you fill-out the FREE Order Forms.

Testimonials!

I thought you might like to know what a few of my customers think about my Survival Products. So here are a couple testimonials from a some of my many testimonials.

This first testimonial is from South Africa. This married couple purchased the Flag Ship of my Survival Products, the 60-pound *2012 Ultra-Advanced Anytime Anywhere Survival Program TOTAL Package (2012 U-AASPTP)*. Some of my subscribers are already survival experts in their own right and in this case, this couple ventures into the African wilderness where they are already in the food-chain. There are NO sissy white-tailed deer over there. They are both highly educated (Wallace has a Ph.D. - Doctorate) and both are survival experts in the African wilderness. It was a challenge for me to put a quality Survival Product in front of these 'African survival experts.'

*"Joseph, I can make fire in at least 40 ways. However, you have managed to learn an old dog some new tricks. Joseph, the subjects covered in your news letters, is extremely interesting, researched in depth, and very relevant to the subject of survival, **it stimulates the reader to think lateral**. Joseph, I am impressed with the time and effort you have put into the practical side of your survival program.*

*There are very few view people who actually test things before they publish it, especially to the extent you do I can't stop reading, every day something new is added to my knowledge. Joseph, I have them all (the books, courses, videos and kits), it's my passion survival and bush skills. **Your program... has proven practical information – THE BEST OF THEM ALL – FOR SURE.**"*
Wallace V. – South Africa – 15 May 2006

This second testimonial is from a wise subscriber. When I first read the testimonial, I chuckled. But when I re-read it several more times, I finally understood what Richard was really telling me. It's a GREAT COMPLIMENT & TESTIMONIAL from Richard.

*"Your organization was exemplary. **This is indeed the best course I have ever spent any money on, and I have bought many**. If this material was taught to all military personal we would be unstoppable. **RAMBO WISHES HE HAD YOU AS A TEACHER**. Your newsletters let me feel like I am in class, even while on a train, plain, or bus. Your videos are the next best thing if one is not physically there. Every American needs to know this material."*
Richard L. E., Boston - 06 Sep. 2001

Note: Even though Rambo is a bad ass fictional character, do you see what he's trying to say about the Rambo comment?

And this third Testimonial is from Scott, and it is blunt and to the point and compares my Survival Programs against the other Survival books, courses, programs,…. out there. See *"About The Author."*

*"Yes, simply outstanding. This really is a Total Package – professional. **The problem with other programs is amatures training amatures = amatures**. Not so with the Anytime Anywhere Survival Program TOTAL Package (AASPTP). If you want to get past the fantasy & Walter Mitty crap & learn the real life down & dirty survival info **this one is it** (U-AAASPTP). **The survival & fire starting tricks is priceless**."*
Scott H., Oklahoma - 24 Jan. 2001

For more Testimonials see www.suvivalexpertbooks.com

Private Mailing List - Order Form - A!

THANK YOU for your very wise interest in my survival work. I promise you I'll give you more than you expect. You'll surely get your money's worth.

My long time philosophy when it comes to teaching international survival is that you're learning from the **REAL SURVIVORS** throughout the globe and throughout history. Here's a partial list of the **REAL SURVIVORS** at www.survivalexpertbooks.com (see *The Real Survivors*)

To send you your choice of Survival Tricks described on the previous pages, I need your permission.

Simply mark (**X**) your choice of Survival Tricks. Before you mark your choices, did you go to **www.survivalexpertbooks.com/private-list**? <u>I have a BONUS waiting for you!!</u>

01) _____ PRSC   06) _____ Emergency Fire-Starting…

02) _____ Sauna In A Can   07) _____ Panamanian Fishing…

03) _____ Home Invasion Defense   08) _____ 100% Weather Forecaster

04) _____ Laydon's Burn/Pain Remedy…   09) _____ Goose Final Approach

05) _____ Snakebite/Spider Remedy…   10) _____ No Weapon Duck Hunting

<u>This is **NOT** an E-Mail offer</u>. I will send everything as promised via the good ol' United States Post Service. And I'll send everything via First Class Mail.

Again, this is a **FREE OFFER**. I will send you your choice of Survival Tricks and I WON'T HOLD BACK! You'll get every single word – the full complete details & sketches.

Why am I doing this? I hope to gain your trust so I can send you *"35 International Survival Tricks"* (really 100+ Survival Tricks) for the price of fast food meal.

And even if you decide not to get *"35 International Survival Tricks"*, I'm very confident the Survival Tricks you pick out today will greatly enhance your self-reliance so You're Ready Anytime Anywhere for decades in the future.

NO, I'm not sending you some crap info. In my humble opinion, your choice of Survival Tricks are very worthy of your attention. I'll send EVERYTHING, FREE, as advertised.

To get your choice of Survival Tricks, all you have to do is mark (**X**) your choices above, fill-out the Order Form (both pages) and send them to me. **DO NOT** send me any money. Like I've stated multiple times, this is a **FREE OFFER** to introduce you to my survival work starting in September 1991 to the present day (**www.survivalexpert.com**).

Private Mailing List - Order Form - B!

Fill-out the Order Form below and send it back to me.
I'll get your Survival Tricks in the mail real quick.
I'll send them to you via First Class Mail.

YES Joseph, send me my choice of Survival Tricks. I
understand there is **NO CHARGE** for the Survival Tricks.
I'm sending this Order Form to you today.

_____

PRINT Last Name   First   MI / Jr. Sn.

_____

Street Address   / P.O. Box   Apt.

_____

City   State   Zip Code

_____

YOUR SIGNATURE   I AM 21+ Years Of Age Or 17+ (Active Duty USA Military and
Allies). I understand these Survival Tricks are 'For Information Use Only.' I understand I will
keep this information confidential and will not share this information. I understand this
Survival Information is protected under Unites States of America Copyright Laws.

SEND Order Form Pages To:
Joseph A. Laydon Jr. (IRISAP)
P.O. Box 48
Cutler, IL 62238-0048
United States of America
          IRISAP Copyright - All Rights Reserved - 2017